The PE... ...... for Women Over 50

Written for Senior Women, perfect for all!

TWO MANUSCRIPT

KETO FOR WOMEN OVER 50

INTERMITTENT FASTING FOR WOMEN OVER 50

JULIA CHRISTEN

TABLE OF CONTENTS

Book 1: Keto for women over 50

Book 2: Intermittent Fasting for women over 50

Keto for Women Over 50

JULIA CHRISTEN

Introduction

The following chapters will discuss exactly how easy it is to lose weight and maintain a healthy weight even after age fifty. The old saying is that age is just a number, and in most cases, it is, but women who are past age fifty know that this old saying is not exactly true. Once the woman has reached age fifty, her body goes through changes that are perfectly normal and perfectly aggravating at the same time! But this is an exciting time for a woman to be alive. This time is the time when many women finally come into their own space and begin to live life for themselves and what better way to do that than by taking control of your body and your health?

This book has all the answers you need to help you to do all of that. Once you understand the changes your body is going through and how to address these changes, you will begin to live the full, rich life that you deserve to live. Health and beauty begin on the inside, and this book will show you exactly how to get started on the changes that will carry you through the next chapter of your life.

There are plenty of books on this subject on the market, thanks again for choosing this one! Every effort was made to ensure it is full of as much useful information as possible, and please enjoy!

Chapter One

WHAT IS THE KETOGENIC DIET?

As far back as the ancient physicians in Greece, we have been told that healthy weight can easily be maintained by restricting the intake of calories from food. For centuries people fasted to treat various illnesses, particularly epilepsy. In the early twentieth century, doctors began experimenting with fasting as a way to control the effects of epilepsy, in the days before medications were introduced. It was found that people who subscribed to the 'water diet' had fewer seizures and were sometimes considered 'cured.' As you can probably guess the water diet consisted of water. And while people did enjoy a respite from seizures it is difficult to maintain a healthy lifestyle while consuming a diet made up of only water.

But this was an exciting time for medical discoveries as patients and physicians alike were beginning to wonder exactly what made the bodywork the way it did. An endocrinologist discovered that people who lived on the water diet secreted three compounds from their livers that were water-soluble, meaning they were flushed away by water. These three compounds together were called 'ketones.'

Since it was impossible to live on water for the remainder of a person's life, doctors began experimenting with different combinations of food so that their epileptic patients could eat. They discovered that a diet that was lower in carbohydrates and rich in fats with a good amount of protein would produce the same epilepsy-free results that the water diet did. Patients could consume a diet of specific foods that mimicked the effect of fasting on their bodies. Eating more fat and removing sugar from the diet caused the liver to release the ketones that the body would then use for energy. Physicians had already concluded that the ketones the body was releasing were the main cause of epileptic seizures and since these were also released by the liver on a high-fat low carb diet, they named this diet the ketogenic diet.

So, physicians used this diet with great success on children and adults who had epilepsy. Seizures lessened or stopped altogether, and people were able to resume a normal life. But then doctors began noticing that people who followed the keto diet, the children especially, were displaying other changes in their bodies that went beyond the cessation of seizures. These people lost weight and were more active. They slept better at night and were more alert during the day. The children especially were easier to discipline and much less irritable than before.

But eventually, anticonvulsant drugs were invented that allowed people with epilepsy to take medication and be free from the restrictions of the dietary plan. This reversal of thought was during a time when refrigeration was still not widely used so that following the constraints of the keto diet may have been difficult for many people. And taking a pill was so much easier. So, the keto diet was no longer taught in medical school and generally fell out of favor with most doctors until a prominent event in the latter part of the twentieth century that changed the way people looked at keto and brought it into the modern world.

At that time a television producer and his wife were looking for something to help their young son who suffered from severe seizures. Even strong medications would not control the child's seizures that would often come one after the other. While doing internet research, his parents stumbled over a description of the ketogenic diet, which would eventually revolutionize their lives. When they started their young son on the keto diet, his seizures virtually vanished, and he was finally able to enjoy life as a normal little boy. A made-for-tv movie soon followed, and the world was once again in love with the keto diet.

But even with its success in treating epilepsy, the keto diet would not have been thought of so favorably if it did not help people to achieve and maintain a normal healthy weight. And while the keto diet itself is relatively new, this style of eating has been around since the time of early man. Hunting and gathering was a way of life for our ancient ancestors. They hunted meat and gathered plants and berries as they traveled from place to place hunting meat. And no part of the meat was wasted, which meant that early man also ate the fat part of the meat along with the lean part. As each generation has moved less and relied on processed foods more, we have gradually become more obese and less healthy.

Enter the keto diet. Following the keto diet relies on a heavy intake of fats, a moderate intake of protein, and a low intake of carbohydrates to achieve weight loss and later to maintain a healthy weight. The main function of the keto diet is to put your body into a state of ketosis which will then cause your body to produce ketones that your body will use for energy instead of using the sugar from the foods that you consume. A high carbohydrate diet will repress the ability of the body to produce ketones, and the excess sugar gets stored as fat.

When you eat the food that you consume goes into your stomach where acids and enzymes mix with the chewed food and help to break it down into even smaller particles. When your meal leaves your stomach, it has been liquified for easier passage into and through the small intestine. In the small intestine, the body completes the job of digesting your food and begins to move it into your bloodstream to other parts of the body. While your gall bladder produces bile to help digest your food and your liver stores nutrients and filters out toxins, your pancreas is perhaps the next most important organ in the food use process. The pancreas is the main organ in your body that helps to regulate your blood sugar levels through its production of insulin.

The hormone insulin is made by the pancreas to help your body use glucose (sugar) from the food that you eat for energy. While the body needs this sugar for energy the molecules of sugar do not pass into the cells by themselves. They need to attach to molecules of insulin in order to be able to enter the cells. When you consume food your blood sugar level rises and this triggers the pancreas to release insulin to help carry the sugar into the cells so that the cells can use the sugar for energy. The problem arises when people either eat too much food overall or they eat too many simple carbs that will turn into sugar in the body. When this happens, the body receives too many signals too often for increasing the level of insulin. Eventually, the cells will stop reacting to insulin because they are full of glucose and have no room for more. Then the excess glucose is stored in the body as excess body fat. When this happens you now have two overwhelming problems, insulin resistance, and obesity.

Many older women have a problem with excess belly fat, and the reason for this is simple. Excess glucose is stored as fat in the body, and the body will search for the easiest place to dump this glucose. The cavities of the midsection, around the internal organs in the abdomen, are the perfect place – in the opinion of the body – to dump off all of that excess sugar so it can turn into fat. The insulin turns the glucose into glycogen and stores it in your belly for possible future needs.

So, it is a known fact that eating more food than you really need for survival leads to obesity. By continuously overeating we train our bodies to think that they need food all day long, which simply is not true. Many cultures around the world discourage snacking between meals and those people tend to live long healthy lives. So, we keep overeating and then one day we realize that we have a body that is filled with little pockets of fat. You will need to rid your body of this excess fat by exercising regularly and consuming a healthy diet. And this is where the keto diet will be the most beneficial.

While we refer to keto as the 'keto diet' it should not really be thought of as a diet. No one should ever plan to live on a diet forever, as that implies restricting things and we do not like to deprive ourselves. Rather, keto should be thought of as a way of life that you will follow in order to make yourself be healthy and fit. When you live the keto way of life your body will start by breaking down excess fat and using these reserves for energy. This is what the body does naturally during times of starvation; it uses stored fat to fuel the body when new food sources are not readily available.

But won't any diet plan work for that purpose? No, not really. Remember that the woman's body naturally stores an extra bit of fat in case we get pregnant. We need to have enough energy in reserve to feed the growing baby. And this is exactly why a man and a woman will have drastically different results on the same diet. The man will lose weight while the woman probably won't and might even gain weight. When a man cuts calories his body turns to stored fat reserves. When a woman cuts calories her metabolism slows down.

The keto diet does not care if you are male or female because it works the same way on everybody. The keto diet restricts carb intake to a level that forces the liver to produce ketones that cause the body to burn stored fat for fuel. The liver naturally produces ketones, just not at the level that it does during ketosis. The liver stores glucose as glycogen and the body will fill up the liver before it fills up any other space in the body. When the body is deprived of substantial carbohydrate intake it turns to the glycogen in the liver to produce energy for the functions of the cells. Since the liver can only store about forty-eight hours with glycogen for energy it must then turn to outside sources like belly fat. When your liver is depleted of stored glycogen and begins to take stores from the body to metabolize for energy then you have entered the state of ketosis.

Do not confuse ketosis with ketoacidosis which is a harmful condition brought on as a result of Type 1 Diabetes.

Ketosis comes on anywhere from two days to one week after beginning the keto diet. This is the goal of the keto diet, to push your body into ketosis. Once you have reached a state of ketosis you will need to maintain the diet in order to remain in ketosis. Getting into ketosis is the worst side effect of the keto diet but once you get past the initial stage you will not regret your decision. Ketosis is often referred to as keto flu because the symptoms feel much like you have viral flu. The symptoms of beginning ketosis are varied:

- Sleep disturbances
- Exhaustion
- Headaches
- Irritability and moodiness
- Bad breath

- Weakness during exercise and after
- Constipation
- Bloating
- Cravings for sugary foods
- Temporary loss of libido
- Diarrhea

The bad breath of ketosis is caused by waste products being eliminated from your body. These waste products are stored in fat cells and need to be eliminated as the fat cells are eliminated. Your body will eliminate waste through your breath, your sweat, or through defecation or urination.

You might naturally feel deprived of sugary treats when you begin the keto diet. We all love a good glazed doughnut or a huge bowl of cake and ice cream and we miss these when they are gone. Just remember they are not gone forever and there are plenty of satisfying dessert options on the keto diet. You will crave carbs because they taste good, but you will be consuming enough foods so that you will not need the carbs to make up for the caloric intake. And decreasing carb intake may lead to a decrease in your ability to get a good night's sleep. Consuming carbs causes the brain to release hormones melatonin and serotonin which are the hormones that make you sleepy and happy respectively. Eventually, the keto diet will teach your body to release hormones at the proper times but in the meantime try to keep a consistent sleep schedule even on your days off.

Some people will experience bloating, constipation, or diarrhea when beginning the keto diet. Food affects all people differently. Diarrhea comes from the increase in fats in your diet. The bloating is from the body releasing toxins from the stored fats that are being digested. Constipation may also go along with increased urination. Fat cells are the primary sources of water storage in your body. When you begin eliminating fat cells the excess water leaves your body in the form of perspiration or urination, leaving very little for the bowels to use for defecation. And less water in your body may lead to feelings of fatigue or muscle weakness.

Moodiness and irritability come from the fact that you are now consuming fewer carbs than before. Carbs almost immediately turn into sugar when they are consumed, and this is true whether the carb is a honey bun or a potato. The body does not care about the difference in healthy or unhealthy food, it just cares that food is coming in. Excess levels of sugar in the blood cause the body to release the hormones dopamine and serotonin which make you calm and happy. This is also why people often fall asleep after consuming a meal that is full of carbs. Removing these foods means that the brain will not signal the release of these hormones and you might feel irritable or moody for a few days.

High-fat diets will increase the level of estrogen in the woman's body because estrogen is stored in fat. So, the more estrogen you have in your body the higher your desire for sexual activity will be, and this is often lost during the first days of ketosis as all of those stored fat cells begin to disappear. When the body has eliminated enough stored fat and has begun functioning at a proper level then the hormone levels will balance themselves out, the estrogen production will return to normal, and your sex drive will reappear.

While these all might seem like good reasons to avoid the keto diet altogether, remember that these side effects are temporary and the beneficial effects of the keto diet are permanent. There are things that you can do to combat the effects of the keto flu and the beginning of ketosis to help you get through this period:

- Drink plenty of water to stay hydrated
- Add sea salt to your water to help ease muscle cramps. Lemon juice will help mask the saltiness
- Engage in gentle exercises like walking, bicycling, or swimming
- Chew gum or suck mints that are sugar-free
- Get a regularly scheduled seven to nine hours of sleep every night

Focusing on the positive benefits of the keto diet may also help you get through ketosis. The keto diet will naturally promote weight loss and assist you with managing your weight. You can easily incorporate the keto diet into your regular lifestyle. Fats and proteins will make you feel full for a longer time so you will eventually consume less food. Food cravings will disappear and hunger will be eliminated. There is really no need to count calories on the keto diet unless you are going for a specific weight loss goal. Keto will not slow down your metabolism so you will continue to lose weight even after the first few weeks on the diet. You will feel more energetic and will be able to better focus on everyday tasks. Your muscles will become stronger and leaner.

Keto flu fades away and you are left with the positive side effect of the keto diet which will last your entire lifetime. All bodies are different and you may not see the same results that your neighbor might enjoy on the same diet plan. But follow the diet, eat the right foods, and you will be successful.

Chapter Two

CHANGES IN YOUR BODY
AFTER AGE 50

If you have reached age fifty, then you should congratulate yourself. You have been through school, teen years, relationships, children, and most importantly the changing of your body. You might be looking at your body and asking it exactly what happened during the last few years. Some things you have not been able to control, like hereditary medical issues and the ravage that time puts on our bodies. Accidents and illnesses are also beyond our control. But you can begin now to understand the changes in your body and make plans to reduce or eliminate as many of the negative changes as you possibly can.

The first thing that will probably happen to you is the onset of menopause. The most notable thing about menopause is that your monthly periods will stop – forever! Menopause is the biggest single change that your body will ever experience besides puberty. Menopause can lead to belly fat, weight gain, and osteoporosis. It is a natural occurrence in the life of every woman, caused by the body making less of the hormones estrogen and progesterone.

Estrogens (there are more than one) is the name for the group of sex-related hormones that make women be women. They cause and promote the initial development and further maintenance of female characteristics in the human body. Estrogens are what gave you breasts, hair in the right places, the ability to reproduce, and your monthly cycle. Estrogen is the hormone that does all of the long-term work in maintaining femininity. Progesterone has one purpose in the woman's body, and that is to implant the egg in the uterus and keep her pregnant until it is time to deliver the baby.

In women, estrogen is crucial to becoming and remaining womanly. In the ovaries, it stimulates the growth of eggs for reproduction. It causes the vagina to grow to a proper adult size. Estrogen promotes the healthy growth of the fallopian tubes and the uterus. And it causes your breasts to grow and to fill with milk when the baby is coming. Estrogen is also responsible for making women store some excess fat around their thighs and hips. This weight storage is nature's way of ensuring that the baby will have nutrition during times of famine.

One of the forms of estrogen dramatically decreases in production after menopause, and this form helps women to regulate the rate of their metabolism and how fast they gain weight. After menopause women tend to gain more weight in their middle area of the body, in the abdomen. This fat collects around the organs and is known as visceral fat. Besides being unattractive visceral fat is also dangerous, because it has been linked to some cancers, heart disease, stroke, and diabetes.

But a lack of estrogen is not the only reason women tend to gain weight after age fifty. Besides a lack of estrogen, the biggest single reason that women over fifty gain weight is lifestyle changes. They are no longer running children to activities; so many women move less after fifty. And sometimes they move less because their joints have begun to ache. Stiffness begins to set in, especially in the morning when rolling out of bed suddenly becomes a chore. Many continue to cook large meals and have difficulty scaling back to cooking for just one or two people, and someone needs to eat that food. And some women still feel that life ends when the children leave so they might as well just indulge a little.

14

But all of this indulging and relaxing leads to loss of muscle strength, loss of flexibility, and increased belly fat, which in turn leads to even more problems. It also leads to an increase in osteoporosis. The lack of estrogen is the leading cause of osteoporosis, which translates literally to the porous bone. The bones in the body, particularly the long bones of the arms and the legs, become more porous as the quality and density of the bone is reduced. Bones will continue to regrow and refresh themselves all of your life, but in osteoporosis, the bone is deteriorating faster than new growth can replace it.

Estrogen helps to decrease overall cholesterol levels in young women which is why women sometimes remain healthy even when they don't take the time to eat healthy meals. All of these changes after fifty and the arrival of menopause because suddenly the estrogen levels drop dramatically. This increase in cholesterol in the body can lead to strokes and heart attacks. Cholesterol is a substance that occurs naturally in your body and is made by the liver. Cholesterol in your body also comes from the foods that you eat. The two kinds that your doctor will measure with a blood test are high-density lipoprotein (HDL) and low-density lipoprotein (LDL). The two numbers together make up your total cholesterol number. Estrogen promotes HDL and depresses LDL, so a lack of estrogen will allow for a higher LDL number.

HDL is the type of cholesterol known as the good type because it removes excess amounts of cholesterol from your arteries and then carries it to the liver where it can be metabolized and removed from the body during waste removal. LDL is the bad form of cholesterol because it likes to sit in your arteries and form deposits known as plaque. It is possible to have a high total cholesterol number and still be considered healthy if the number is high because the HDL is high and the LDL is low. This means that your body is doing the right thing and the good cholesterol is eliminating the bad cholesterol.

When LDL clumps in the arteries and forms plaques it causes hardening of the arteries. Blood will not flow very well through stiff arteries. Your heart will need to work harder to push the blood through your body. And if you have gained a significant amount of weight your body has created new arteries to supply blood flow to this increased part of you. This will also make the heart work harder than it needs to. And if plaque builds up in the arteries that are connected to the heart those arteries can become clogged which results in coronary artery disease. This can cause a heart attack if a piece of plaque breaks loose and cuts off the steady flow of blood to the muscles of the heart. If this happens in the arteries that lead to the brain it can cause a stroke.

Too much cholesterol has also been found in the brains of people who suffered from Alzheimer's disease. And an excessive amount of cholesterol can cause gallstones, which women are naturally at a higher risk of anyway.

You may have noticed that you seem to be losing control of your bladder function, or that laughing or sneezing makes you dribble a bit. This is also a normal effect of aging because the muscles just are not as strong as they used to be. Also, the excess weight pressing down on the bladder does not help the situation.

While it is impossible to stop the process of aging there are things every woman can do to slow the process and help her body remain healthy far into the future. One of the most important ways women can do this is to maintain a healthy weight, which is what makes the keto diet is so important to all women and especially to those over age fifty.

Chapter Three

USING KETO TO CONTROL OR PREVENT AGE-RELATED CONDITIONS

Everyone gradually gets older. It is an undeniable fact of life. But even though we are aging all of the time, we do not need to be old, not yet anyway. It is possible to be an active, vibrant woman at fifty and beyond if you make some smart choices and take care of yourself. And deciding to follow the keto way of life is the smartest choice you could have made. The keto diet isn't just good for weight loss, although that is probably its most important and noticeable feature. The keto diet gives so much more to your body while it is helping you to lose and then maintain your weight.

The keto diet will result in increased brain function and the ability to focus. The brain normally uses sugar to fuel its processes, but the consumption of sugar has its own problems. The brain can easily switch to using ketones for fuel and energy. Remember that ketones are the by-product of ketosis that makes you burn fat. And the keto diet was used by doctors to control seizures in patients long before medications were invented. The exact way this works is still not completely understood, but researchers believe it has something to do with the neurons stabilizing as excess sugar is removed from the diet and hormones are better regulated. Patients with Alzheimer's disease have been seen to have increased cognitive function and enhanced memory when they consume a keto diet. And these same changes in the chemical makeup of the brain can lead to fewer migraines overall and less severe migraines.

When the keto diet helps you to lose weight, it also helps you to reduce your risk of cardiovascular disease. These diseases include anything that pertains to the cardiovascular system, which means heart attacks, strokes, plaque formations, peripheral artery disease, blood clots, and high blood pressure. Plaque buildups, which are caused by excess weight and cholesterol, lead to a condition known as atherosclerosis. The plaque will gather in the arteries and form clogs that narrow the artery and restrict the flow of blood. The plaque is formed from fat cells, waste products, and calcium deposits that are found floating in the blood. When you lose weight and decrease the amount of fat and cholesterol in the body there will be less to accumulate in the arteries and the blood will naturally flow better with less restriction.

Being overweight can cause high blood pressure. When the doctor measures the force of your blood pressure as it moves through your arteries, he is measuring your blood pressure. If you are overweight your heart will need to push the blood harder to get it through the increased lengths of arteries it had to create in order to feed your cells. And if there is a buildup of plaque in the arteries then the heart will need to push the blood harder to get it past the blockage. This, in turn, creates thin spots in the arteries which is a good place for plaque to build up. Since this condition comes on gradually over the course of years as you slowly gain weight it gives off no immediate symptoms and that is why it is often referred to as the silent killer. Strokes and heart attacks are caused by unchecked high blood pressure.

The single most important way to control high blood pressure is to control your weight. You can't change the family history but you can control your weight and your lifestyle. Since high blood pressure is caused by the heart needing to work harder than the act reducing the strain on the heart will cause it to work less strenuously in bad ways. Losing weight and maintaining a healthy weight will ease the strain on your heart. If the blood pressure is not pumping too high then it will not cause weak spots in your arteries. If there are no weak spots then there is no place for plaque to collect. And if there is no excess fat or cholesterol in the blood there will be no plaque formations to collect in the blood.

A diet that is high in saturated fats is a risk factor for heart disease. While keto is a high-fat diet it is high in monounsaturated fats. Polyunsaturated and monounsaturated fats are good for you while trans fats and saturated fats are not. Mono – and polyunsaturated fats are the good fats that are found in fatty fish like salmon and in certain plants like avocados, olives, and certain seeds and nuts that are all staples of the keto diet. Saturated fats and trans fats are found in breaded deep-fried foods, baked goods, processed foods, and pre-packaged snack foods like popcorn. When your doctor measures your LDL and HDL he also measures your level of triglycerides, which is a type of fat that is found floating in the bloodstream and that is responsible for elevating the risk of heart attacks, especially in women over fifty. Reducing the number of saturated fats and trans fats that you consume will automatically reduce the amounts of triglycerides floating in your blood.

Inflammation is a part of life, especially for women over the age of fifty. There are good kinds of inflammation, such as when white blood cells rush to a particular body area to kill an infection. But mostly older women are plagued by the bad forms of inflammation which make your joints swell and cause early morning stiffness. Carrying too much weight on your body will cause inflammation and pain in the joints, especially in the lower part of the body where the weight-bearing joints like the knees and the hips are located. When a joint feels pain it sends a signal to the brain that there is a pain, and the body sends cells to combat that pain. The helper cells don't know there really isn't anything wrong but they come prepared to fight and this causes inflammation around the joint. One extra pound of excess weight will put four pounds of pressure on the knee joints. Losing weight will help to eliminate inflammation in the body. And cutting down on the intake of carbs will help to lessen the amount of inflammation in the body because carbs cause inflammation. Decreasing the inflammation in your body will also help to eliminate acne, eczema, arthritis, psoriasis, and irritable bowel syndrome.

Adopting the keto way of life will also help to eliminate problems with the kidneys and improve their function. Kidney stones and gout are caused mainly by the elevation of certain chemicals in the urine that helps to create uric acid which is what we eliminate in the bathroom. The excess consumption of carbohydrates and sugar will lead to a buildup of calcium and phosphorus in your urine. This buildup of excess chemicals can cause kidney stones and gout. When your ketones begin to raise the acid in your urine will briefly increase as your body begins to eliminate all of the waste products from the fats that are being metabolized, but after that, the level will decrease and will remain lower than before as long as you are on the keto diet.

Eating a diet that is high carb can eventually cause problems with your gallbladder including gallstones. These stones are little deposits of hardened fluid that get trapped in your gallbladder and cause great pain. The gallbladder is built to release bile into the small intestine to help digest the food that you eat. When the liver produces more cholesterol than your gallbladder can produce bile to digest, the excess cholesterol forms stones in the gallbladder.

Eating a low carb diet will eliminate much of the excess cholesterol that your liver produces and the high fat of the keto diet will help the gallbladder to cleanse itself.

Vegetables that grow in the ground, grain-based foods, processed foods, and sugary foods all contribute to heartburn and acid reflux by raising the level of acid in the stomach. There is a band of muscles that is wound tightly around the bottom of your esophagus, the muscular tube that takes food from your mouth to your stomach. This band of muscles is called the esophageal sphincter. It will relax just enough to let food pass into the stomach when it is healthy. But a constant diet of the wrong kinds of foods will increase the stomach acid, which in turn washes over this sphincter and eventually weakens it, which allows stomach acid to flow backward and up into the esophagus. Eating the low carb keto diet will improve the acid reflux symptoms and will help to relieve the inflammation of the esophagus and the stomach.

The best overall benefit of the keto lifestyle is the fact that it will lower your overall weight, which will have a positive effect on your entire body. Lower weight will mean freedom from the effects of obesity which can help to get rid of metabolic syndrome and Type 2 Diabetes. The condition known as Metabolic Syndrome happens when the body becomes resistant to insulin and the insulin your body produces is no recognized by the cells in your body. This is what causes the body to store your excess blood sugar as fat in your body, especially around the area of the stomach. When you begin the keto diet and enter ketosis the body will be forced to use these fat stores for energy and the body's production of insulin will be returned to normal. The amount of protein in the diet will help your muscles keep their strength and tone and not begin to wither as so often happens in older women.

Following the keto diet will mean that you will eat less food but it will be more filling and more nutritious. When you eat fats and proteins instead of carbs you will feel fuller much longer with less food. Lowering your caloric intake will help you lose weight and less weight will make you healthier. It will also slash your risk of developing certain diseases and will minimize the effects of others. These are the life improvements that the keto lifestyle has to offer you.

Chapter Four

FOOD LIST FOR KETO EATING

I f you have done any reading on the keto diet or heard other people talking about it. If so, you may have heard the term 'macros.' It sounds like a magical, mystical term that goes along with this new magical diet plan. People who have lived the keto lifestyle for a while love to share their knowledge, and some of it is very good. But there is a huge difference of opinion when it comes to the macros.

Macros are nothing more than a shortened version of the word macronutrient. A macronutrient is a component of the food that you use to fuel your body. In other words, a macro is a fat, protein, or carbohydrate. In the opinion of some people, you need to track your macros in order to make certain that you are getting the correct balance of nutrients. And some people feel that you do not need to track your macros as long as you correctly follow the guidelines for the keto diet that pertain to avoiding carbs and eating a high-fat diet.

On a standard keto diet, you will consume a diet that is five percent carbohydrates, twenty to twenty-five percent proteins, and seventy-five percent fats. If you are counting your macros then you will need to decide how many calories you want to consume in one day, and then you will need to multiply your food percentages by your total calories to see how many calories of each macro you can eat in one day. The calculation would look something like this:

2000 calorie diet

$$2000 \times 5\% \text{ carbs} = 100 \text{ grams of carbs}$$

$$2000 \times 20\% \text{ proteins} = 400 \text{ grams of proteins}$$

$$2000 \times 75\% \text{ fats} = 1500 \text{ grams of fats}$$

The key is in knowing exactly what is in your food. So, on the keto diet, you will either read a lot of food labels or you will be making most of your food from scratch. The number of calories that you choose to consume will depend on many factors such as your height, activity level, and how much weight you want to lose.

You will notice that the ratio of carbs on the keto diet is very low. There are good reasons for this. Carbs turn directly to sugar when they are consumed, and the type of carb does not matter; eventually, they all will produce some amount of sugar in your body during digestion. A complex carb, such as a potato or a beet, will take longer to digest and will make less sugar than a sweet roll or a slice of bread, but they all turn out the same way. Also, there is no real essential carbohydrate. There are essential amino acids (proteins) and fatty acids (fats), but there are no carbs that you must eat in order to maintain a healthy lifestyle.

When you are reading food labels or recipe information there is a particular way to know how many net carbs are in the food that you are eating. So look on a nutrition label and find the line that says 'total carbs.' Then find the line that says 'fiber.' Fiber is considered a carb but it does not count toward your total carb intake because fiber passes through your body as waste because it is not digestible. So, you will subtract the amount of fiber from the total carbs number to decide your net carb count, like this:

$$17 \text{ grams of carbs} - 5 \text{ grams of fiber} = 12 \text{ grams of net carbs}$$

Net carbs are the starches and sugars that are leftover when the fiber count is removed. This is the number that you will count toward your daily allowance of carbs. You will need to know which foods are low in carbs and which ones you should eat rarely or never. And when you are looking for those added carbs on your food labels you want to look for glucose, sucrose, dextrose, fructose, galactose, maltose, cellulose, dextrin, glycogen, and any word that ends in saccharide. Words to look for that will alert you to the added presence of added sugar are cane sugar, corn sugar, brown sugar, confectioner's sugar, beet sugar, beetroot, grape sugar, dextrose, fruit sugar, levulose, maltose, malt sugar, lactose, milk sugar, invert sugar, maple sugar, and saccharose.

When you think about the foods that are allowed on the keto diet you might begin to think that the keto diet is the most restrictive diet you have ever seen. In one way it is because you will not be allowed to eat those sugary treats you might be so fond of. But there are plenty of tasty carbs that are allowed on the keto diet, and they are carbs that are good for your body. Some will say that everything that you eat should be organic and fresh. Meat should be grass-fed or free-range, eggs should come from free-range chickens and cheese should be made from the milk of grass-fed cows. While this is nice it just isn't necessary. Organic food is usually more expensive than similar non-organic food and it may not be easily available where you live. And not all food should be purchased fresh. If you live in a city with open-air markets or you like going to the grocery store several times each week then you can buy all of your food fresh. But for most people, this just is not realistic. Canned or frozen food is perfectly fine for the purposes of the keto diet. You will lose weight and eat good food on the keto diet whether it is organic or the same stuff everyone else eats.

So, what are you allowed to eat on the keto diet? Well, there are actually a great many foods that are allowed for keto dieters. You will eat meat, fish, seafood, vegetables, dairy items, fruits, and high-quality fats.

Fish and seafood are rich in the B vitamins as well as selenium and potassium. They are also rich in protein and carbohydrate-free. They are also great sources of Omega-3 fats which will help to increase your sensitivity to insulin and will help to lower the levels of sugar in your blood. You should eat fish and seafood at least two to three times each week.

Nutritional information per three-ounce serving without skin:

FOOD	CALORIES	PROTEIN	CARBS	FAT
Catfish	120	19	0	5
Clams, steamed, 12	120	22	4	2
Cod	90	19	0	1
Flounder	100	20	0	1
Haddock	90	20	0	1
Lobster	100	20	1	1
Mackerel	190	21	0	12
Perch	100	20	0	2
Orange Roughy	70	16	0	1
Oysters, steamed, 12	120	12	7	4
Pollock	100	21	0	1
Rainbow Trout	130	22	0	4
Salmon	150	22	0	7
Scallops, broiled, 14 small	150	29	2	1
Shrimp	110	22	0	2
Sole	100	21	0	1
Whiting	100	19	0	1

Meat and poultry are stapling items on the keto diet and excellent sources of protein. They are generally carb-free and are good sources of the B vitamins as well as the minerals zinc, selenium, and potassium. Bacon and sausage are processed meats that are allowed on the keto diet but they are sources of certain items that might raise your risk for cancer, so limit them whenever possible. Hot dogs and smoked sausage are also good choices but make sure to check the label and look for added sources of sugars or starches.

Here are the nutritional values for three-ounce servings of meats, poultry, and pork:

FOOD	CALORIES	PROTEIN	FAT	CARBS
Beef	220	27	12	0
Chicken, thigh	209	26	10.9	0
Chicken, breast	165	31	3.6	0
Turkey, breast	167	34	2	0
Hot dog, no bun	290	9	23	9
Smoked sausage	210	7	18	4
Pork, tenderloin	125	22	304	0
Pork, cutlet	239	34	10	0
Pork, ground	251	22	18	0
Bacon, one slice	37	3	3	0

The next category in which you will find keto-friendly foods is the dairy department. Certain dairy foods contain a good mix of fats, proteins, and carbs and they are also good sources of Vitamin B-12, calcium, and riboflavin. The nutritional values for the cheese in the following table are for one-ounce servings:

FOOD	CALORIES	CARBS	FATS	PROTEIN
Blue cheese	100	0.7	8.1	6
Brie	95	0.1	7.9	5.9
Cheddar	114	0.4	9.4	7
Cottage cheese	24	1	0.7	3.4
Cream cheese	97	1.2	9.7	1.7

Feta	75	1.2	9.7	1.7
Monterey Jack	106	0.2	8.6	6.9
Mozzarella	85	0.6	6.3	6.3
Parmesan	111	0.9	7.3	10
Swiss	108	1.5	7.9	7.6
Heavy cream, 2 Tbs.	104	0.8	11	0.6
Sour cream, 2 Tbs.	46	0.7	4.7	0.5
Greek yogurt	95	4	5	9
Egg, one	75	0.6	5	7

Vegetables will be your source of carbs and fiber in your diet. These nutritional values are for a one-cup serving unless otherwise noted:

Column1	Column2	Column3	Column4
FOOD	**CARBS**	**FIBER**	**NET CARBS**
Bell peppers	9	3	6
Broccoli	6	2	4
Asparagus	8	4	4
Mushrooms	2	1	1
Zucchini	4	1	3
Spinach, cooked	7	4	3
Spinach, raw	1	1	0
Avocados	13	10	3
Cauliflower	5	3	2
Green beans	10	4	6
Lettuce	2	1	1
Garlic, one cove	1	0.5	0.5
Kale	7	1	6
Cucumbers	4	1	3
Brussels Sprouts	6	2	4
Celery	3	2	1
Tomatoes	6	2	4
Radishes	4	2	2
Onions, one half cup	6	1	5
Eggplant	8	2	6
Cabbage	5	3	2

Artichokes	14	10	4

There are very few fruits that are allowed on the keto diet because the fruit is high in sugar. But the following fruits are allowed and these counts are for a half-cup serving:

FOOD	CARBS	FIBER	NET CARBS
Blackberries	6.9	3.8	3.1
Rhubarb	5.7	4	1.7
Star Fruit	4.4	1.8	2.6
Raspberries	7.3	4	3.3
Cantaloupe	6.8	1	5.8
Strawberries	5.7	1	4.7
Watermelon	6.4	1	5.4
Lemon	2.5	2	0.5
Lime	2.5	2	0.5

You should also stock up on the following food items. These are encouraged for use on the keto diet since some, like broth, will help you to curb hunger between meals and herbs and spices will add flavor to your food without adding carbs or calories. Just remember to look at the label for added starches and sugars:

Olive oil, coconut oil, avocado oil	Lard
Canned fish	Olives, green and black
Sauerkraut	Hot sauce
Flavored water additives, no sugar	Bottled water
Tea	Coffee

Club soda	Herbs and spices
Pork rinds (great for breading foods)	Mayonnaise, full fat
Mustard	Vinegar
Broth	Bouillon cubes

When you go food shopping only buy the things that you know you will eat. That may sound silly but some people will buy a portion of food they do not like just because it is listed on a diet plan. Don't do it! Buy the foods that you want to eat and leave the others for someone else. But also, don't be afraid to try foods you've never tried before or didn't like in the past. The adult you just might like radishes.

It is imperative that you get used to eating real food. Processes food has no place in the life of the keto dieter. Following the keto lifestyle will take more planning than any other diet or meal plan you may have tried, but it is totally worth the effort. Sometimes you might want to cook one large meal and divide it over several days of eating. Many recipes make great leftovers for tomorrow's lunch.

The keto diet does not mean giving up good food or the treats you once indulged in. It does mean making better food choices in order to improve your overall health and well-being. When you begin creating your own menus do not be afraid to experiment with different menu ideas and different ways of putting your food together. You will be pleasantly surprised at just how flexible and how good keto eating really is.

Chapter Five

EXERCISES TO ASSIST WITH QUALITY OF LIFE AFTER 50

The ways that you take care of your body and the ways you stay active will dictate your quality of life and how good you will look. If you do not take care of your body, you might be fifty years old and look like you are sixty-five years old. But if you do good things for your body you might be sixty-five years old and look like you are fifty years old. Age really is just a number. And even if you haven't been active in a long time, or ever, it is never too late to start on some sort of activity plan to increase the quality of your life.

I call it an activity plan because no one really wants to exercise, right? So, let's think of this as an activity plan or a workout routine, both of those are positive statements that say you care about your body and you want to fight the effects of growing older with everything you've got.

Once a woman crosses that fifty-year mark, she begins losing one percent of her muscle each year. But muscle tone and fiber do not need to be lost with aging. With a proper workout, you can continue to build new muscle and maintain what you already have until you are in your nineties. And some of the exercises that you do for your muscles will help you build strong bones. This is especially important for women because losing the estrogen supplies in our bodies will cause us to lose bone mass faster than men do. This is when we are really at risk for developing osteoporosis.

And regular physical activity will help you to avoid developing that middle-age spread around the abdomen or to lose it if you already have it. Activity will help you to maintain a proper weight for your height and build which in turn will help you to avoid many, if not all, of the age-related, obesity-related diseases such as cardiovascular diseases and diabetes.

Physical activity comes in four main types. Each one should be done at least once or twice a week to ensure your body is getting the right mix of activity. The four main types of activity are:

- Balance – Older people lose their sense of balance. It is easy for an older person to fall and break something, like a hip. When you engage in activities that help you to maintain your sense of balance will help reduce the risk that you might fall and suffer a permanent injury.

- Stretching – As we age our muscles begin to lose their elasticity. This is part of why rolling out of bed in the morning gets more difficult as we get older. Stretching activities will help you to improve and maintain your level of flexibility which will help you to avoid injuries to your joints and muscles.

- Cardiovascular/Aerobic – These are also called endurance activities because you should be able to maintain them for at least ten minutes at a time. This key here is to get your heart working faster and your breathing to be deeper. You should be working hard but still able to carry on a conversation. These activities will strengthen your heart and lungs which are, after all, very important muscles in your body.

- Strength training – We are not talking about bodybuilding, but if you want to go for it. This will include working out with resistance bands or lifting weights. Either activity will help to build muscle.

While there are four separate categories of exercise that does not mean that you need to keep them strictly separated because many activities will encompass work in more than one area. You can lift light weights while doing balance activities. Walking and swimming will build muscle strength and cardiovascular health. Yoga will improve balance and assist with building muscle strength and stretching. The key is to engage in seventy-five minutes of vigorous activity each week, or fifteen minutes five days each week; or you can get one hundred fifty minutes of moderate activity in five thirty-minute sessions each week.

And make sure that you design a plan that fits you. Remember that it is perfectly fine to change your routine as your needs change. Maybe, in the beginning, you will work on balance three days each week because you really need help with that. But after a few weeks, your balance has improved enough so that you can devote one of those days to strength training. This is your routine made just for you so make it work for you. And don't forget to get your doctor's okay before beginning any type of activity routine. He will most likely give you his blessings but it is always good to ask. He can also provide you with information on activities that are good for you personally.

One thing to note here, especially if you have not been active in a while, is not to begin a vigorous level of activity the same day you begin the keto diet. During the time your body is getting used to the diet and going through ketosis, you will not feel like indulging in a lot of extra activity and your workout routine will be doomed to failure. This journey is all about making you the best you possibly can so don't sabotage yourself in the first few weeks. If you really want to start your activities on day one of your diet then I recommend walking or bicycling. Either of these activities can be started slowly, so a gentle walk or bike around the neighborhood after dinner is a perfect activity.

If you can get out and join a class at a local senior center, YMCA, community college, or church then do that. You will meet new people, some in your age group, and you can all work together to create your new bodies. But taking a class will not be the best choice for everyone. So we have included some basic exercises that can be done in the privacy of your home to get you started on the new lean you.

STRETCHING – Stretching activities are so important for older adults. These activities will also help you to improve your balance because you might find yourself standing or reaching in new and different ways.

Quad stretch – This is a simple exercise that can be done at home. Hold onto a chair or your partner for balance assistance if you need it. Then with the opposite hand lift the foot on that side behind you. Pull upward gently you can feel the beginning of a stretch in the front of your leg. As people get older, they may lean forward for balance and this muscle, the quad, can become shorter and less efficient over time. Hold this position steady for at least thirty seconds and repeat on the other side.

Hamstring stretch – This activity can be done on the sofa, the bed, or on the floor. Lay one leg in front of you and point your toes to the ceiling. Slowly fold your body over until you feel a stretching in the back of your leg and hold it for thirty seconds.

NOTE: if you have recently had a hip replacement check with your doctor before doing this one.

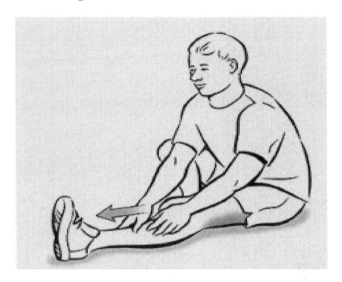

Calf stretch – Place your hands on the wall and step back with one foot. The back foot should be flat on the floor and the front knee should be slightly bent. Then lean forward toward the wall until you feel a stretch in your calf muscle. Hold it for thirty seconds and repeat on the other leg.

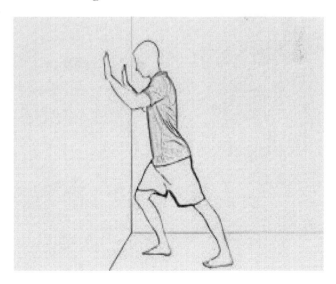

BALANCING – Balancing activities are so important for older adults to reduce the risk of falls. Tai Chi and Yoga are both excellent activities for assisting with better balance. You can find DVDs, routines online, or classes taught by certified instructors. Just remember to work with your body and your current level of ability and don't try to do an advanced routine if you have never mastered a beginner routine. You will just be setting yourself up for failure and we are here to succeed. And keep in mind that flexibility activities also help with the effects of arthritis. While you will want to explore the different types of yoga before making a decision on the one that is best for you, here is a yoga pose that anyone can do at home and helps to wake the whole body in the morning.

Mountain Pose – Stand straight with your feet together. Pull in your stomach muscles as tight as you can and let your shoulders relax. Keep your legs strong but do not lock your knees. Breathe deeply and regularly in and out for ten breaths.

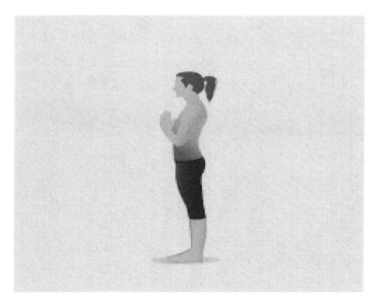

Strength Training – This activity is especially important for you to ensure you keep your muscles strong and healthy for the next phase of your life. You can do many strength training activities without weights, or for an extra challenge add some light hand weights.

Punching – This will strengthen your arms and shoulders and get your blood moving at the same time. Stand straight with your feet apart slightly wider than your shoulders. Keep your stomach firm. Punch straight out with one fist and then the other for at least twenty repetitions.

Squat – This activity is great for strengthening the bottom and the thighs. This will help you to sit down – not fall down – and be able to rise from a seated position with ease and grace. Stand with your feet as far apart as your hips are wide to provide a stable stance. Push your bottom backward as you bend your knees. Your knees should never go out front further than your toes, and try to keep your weight over your heels. If you feel more secure this activity can be done in front of a chair in case you lose your balance and inadvertently sit down.

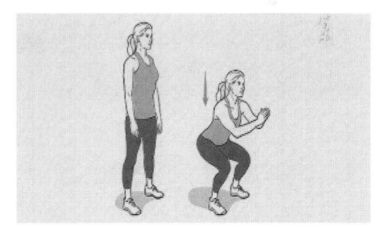

Bridge – Lie on your back with your knees bent and your feet as far apart as your hips. Keep your feet flat on the floor. Pull in your stomach and lift your hips to make a bridge of your back. Hold this pose for ten seconds and try to do at least ten.

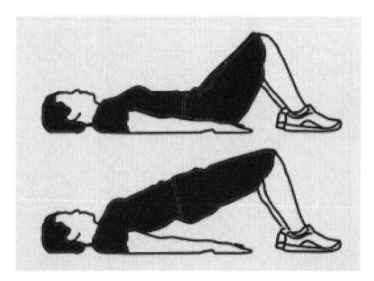

Cardiovascular/Aerobic – The purpose here is to engage in some activity that gets your heart pumping faster and your lungs expanding further. Swimming, walking, running, cycling, aerobics classes, dancing – all of these are great activities for getting the circulation going again. Just remember to begin slowly and pay attention to your body. In other words, if something hurts, stop. But make sure it is really hurt. There is a difference between 'Wow I'm really out of shape because I haven't walked anywhere in a while' and 'My knee really hurts when I do that'. And any time you are ever in doubt seek medical attention.

Seated Activities – The body will deteriorate if it is not used. Maybe you really want to engage in physical activities but you really can't stand up for long enough to do anything meaningful. You can sit down and do many activities that are designed to get you back into the routine of regular movement. Here are a few options for you:

Marching – sit tall in your chair with your feet flat on the floor and your legs bent at a ninety-degree angle. Lift one foot and then the other, as though you are marching in the chair. Raise the knee up in the air and keep the knee bent.

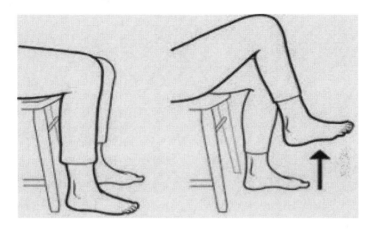

Shoulder Press – Sit tall in your chair. You can hold a set of light weights or simply make your hands into fists. If you do not own weights and do not want to buy any you can also use canned items or full water bottles. Raise your hands up into the air until your arms are straight and then lower them. Do these slowly so that your muscles will actually be doing the work.

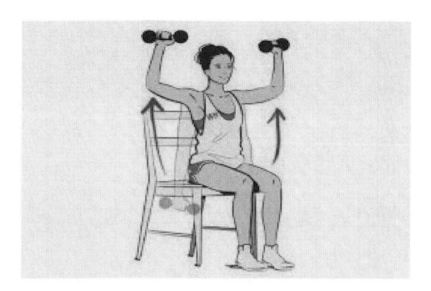

Leg lifts – This activity will strengthen your quads, which is the muscle on the front of your leg. Strong quads are needed for walking upright. Sit tall in your chair with your knees bent at ninety degrees and your feet flat on the floor. Lift a foot up into the air and away from the chair slowly; let the muscle do the work. Hold the pose for five seconds and lower it. Repeat five times on each leg.

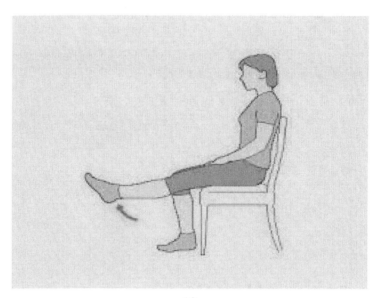

These are just a few of the activities that you can do to get yourself moving and help you in your weight loss and health goals. You are not too old to begin. You can find many routines on the internet so that you can use them alone in the privacy of your home. Remember to preview a routine before you pay for anything in case you do not like it. And many routines are offered free of charge. So do a bit of research and don't stop with one activity. Try to make your routine as varied as possible so that you will not get bored and soon you will have that body you want along with a healthier you.

Chapter Six

STAYING KETO IN REAL LIFE

Once you have spent some time at home preparing your meals and learning the ins and outs of the keto lifestyle, you might be ready to venture out in the real world again. Maybe you have lost some weight and want to debut the new you. Besides, no one really wants to stay home alone every night enjoying their own company. But can you go out in the real world and still remain on the keto diet?

The answer is yes, with a little advance planning and some strategies. Many restaurants now realize that staying relevant and remaining in business means that they will need to adapt their menus to meet the nutritional needs of various people. Simply offering a one-kind-fits-all menu will no longer work in a world where people want or need to eat a particular way and will not accept NO for an answer. And the keto diet is flexible enough that you can find menu options at any eating establishment from fast food to fine dining.

You will want to always look for fish, seafood, meat, and poultry options. Sometimes you can order just the meat portion if the daily veggie is not to your liking. If you are eating the veggie option, make sure it is one from the allowed choices and order a double portion and tell them to hold the potato. Get the salad instead of the soup and specify oil and vinegar dressing on the side. Yes, the bread and rolls will still come to the table to tempt you, but you are strong enough to resist them. If you want to order a burger or a sandwich that is fine but specify that you do not want the bread or the bun. Rice or pasta sides can be replaced by another vegetable. The vinegar and oil dressing for your salad can also be used to season your meat and vegetable options as well as butter. You can also ask for other low carb options like soy sauce, guacamole, hot sauce, vinaigrette, or béarnaise sauce.

You can still eat with friends at a fast-food restaurant. Just ask for your sandwich meat and fixings to be served in a lettuce leaf or in the container without the bun. Do not order onion rings or French fries or hash browns. Top your sandwich with mushrooms, cheese, sprouts, lettuce, bacon, and avocado. Mayonnaise is good, and ketchup is bad. Honey mustard and sweet mustard are bad, but regular yellow mustard is good. Order your chicken grilled, not fried, and have it on a salad. Stay far away from corn, baked beans, sweet potatoes, sweet and sour sauce, and barbecue sauce. A little coleslaw will be fine even though the dressing might be slightly higher in carbs than you really need.

Mexican food restaurants are great for the keto dieter. Keep your hand out of the chip basket. Just because the chips are free does not mean they are good for you. Fill your burrito with shrimp, steak, pork, or chicken and have them serve it in a bowl without the tortilla. Top your choice of meat with the onions and bell peppers used for fajitas. Extra cheese is always a good choice, both for your diet and your taste buds. Use sour cream or salsa to flavor your food. If they won't serve the burrito in a bowl (which is not likely) then just unroll it and eat the insides only. Fajitas, chili verde, carne asada, and chicken mole are all good low carb choices. Tell the server to leave the rice and beans in the kitchen and see if you can get extra sour cream, guacamole, or cheese instead.

The Asian restaurant is not the best choice for the keto dieter. Do not choose any menu item that is battered or has the word 'sweet' in its description. Order the duck without the sauce. Shirataki noodles are low carb and might be your best choice. Other good choices are green beans or sautéed cabbage or sprouts. Stir-fries and curries with low carb veggies are fine but leave the rice in the kitchen.

When you feel adventurous check out a local Indian-themed location. These restaurants are great choices for the keto dieter. Indian cuisine makes regular use of ghee (purified butter) and they put it on everything. Kebabs, curries, meat, and poultry in cream sauce, and Tandoori dishes are all great choices for you. And look for Raita on the menu. It is a creamy dip that is made from yogurt and shredded cucumbers.

One of the best options for a keto dieter is the buffet-style restaurant. You will find dozens of menu items that fit perfectly into your allowed food groups. You should eat to enjoy and don't worry about quantity. Make intentional and deliberate choices, even if it takes you a bit longer to fill up your plate. Your best places to graze will be the salad section and the meat and seafood section. There should be some good choices in the veggies also but stay away from potatoes and rice. And buffets always offer low carb condiments like oil and vinegar, sour cream, cheese, and butter. If the buffet offers sugar-free gelatin have that for dessert.

It is not impossible to follow the keto diet and have fun times with friends. Most restaurants post their menus online and many offers nutritional information. So if you know in advance where you are going you can already have your menu items picked out for when you arrive and order. Just remember that your choices are yours and do not feel the need to eat as others do. You are eating for you and that is the most important choice you will ever make.

Chapter Seven

KETO BREAKFAST RECIPES

The typical breakfast of bacon or ham and eggs is perfect on the keto diet. Just add in cheese and some type of low carb vegetable to round it out into a complete meal.

1.HUEVOS RANCHEROS

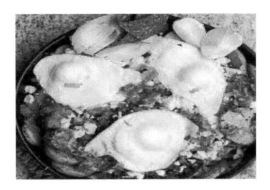

Serves one

Ingredients:

- Cilantro, fresh, one tablespoon
- Yellow onion, one half, chopped
- Avocado, one half
- Garlic, two cloves, minced
- Eggs, two,
- Tomato, one diced
- Salt, one quarter teaspoon
- Black pepper, one teaspoon
- Jalapeno, one fresh, minced
- Orange bell pepper, one half, chopped
- Coconut oil, two tablespoons

Instructions:

Fry the onion, garlic, bell pepper, and jalapeno in half of the coconut oil for five minutes. Pour in the diced tomatoes and fry for an additional five minutes. Beat the eggs in a small bowl and pour over the veggie mix in the skillet, stirring frequently until the eggs are scrambled to desired consistency. Serve with slices of fresh avocado.

Nutrition per serving:

Calories 610, 16 grams net carbs, 51 grams fat, 16 grams protein

2. ITALIAN BREAKFAST CASSEROLE

Serves four

Ingredients:

- Eggs, eight
- Butter, two tablespoons
- Cheddar cheese, five ounces shredded
- Black pepper, one teaspoon
- Salt, one half teaspoon
- Basil, fresh, chopped, one half cup
- Heavy whipping cream, one cup
- Italian sausage, fresh, twelve ounces
- Cauliflower, seven ounces

Instructions

Heat oven to 375. Use lard or oil to grease an eight by eight or nine by nine baking pan. Rinse the cauliflower well and pat it dry, and then chop the cauliflower into small bite-sized pieces. Cook the cauliflower in the melted butter for five minutes, then put it off to the side. Drop the Italian sausage into the skillet and use a firm spatula to chop it up into crumbly pieces. Fry the sausage until it is completely done and dump it into the baking pan with the cauliflower. Beat well together with the pepper, salt, heavy cream, cheddar cheese, and eggs until well mixed. Pour this mixture over the sausage and sprinkle the basil all over the top. Bake the casserole for forty minutes.

Nutrition per serving:

Calories 875, 5 grams net carbs, 79 grams fat, 34 grams protein

3. VEGETARIAN BREAKFAST CASSEROLE

Serves four

Ingredients:

- Eggs, twelve
- Black pepper, one teaspoon
- Salt, one teaspoon
- Onion powder, one teaspoon
- Leek, one half of one
- Green olives, one half cup
- Parmesan cheese, one ounce shredded
- Cherry tomatoes, one half cup
- Shredded cheese, seven ounces
- Heavy whipping cream, one cup

Instructions

Heat oven to 400. Rinse the portion of the leek and trim off the ends, then slice it very thinly. Use lard or oil to grease a thirteen by nine baking pan and lay the leeks in the bottom with the olives. Use a medium-sized bowl to beat together the onion powder, pepper, salt, eggs, cream, and the shredded cheese. Pour all of this mixture over the leeks and olives; do not worry if the leeks and olives move. Top the egg mixture with sprinkles of the parmesan cheese and the cherry tomatoes. Bake for forty minutes.

Nutrition per serving:

Calories 621, 5 grams net carbs, 52 grams fat, 33 grams protein

4. CAULIFLOWER HASH BROWNS

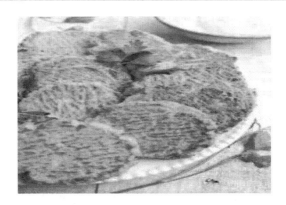

Serves four

Ingredients:

- Eggs, three well beaten
- Butter, four tablespoons
- Yellow onion, one half grated
- Black pepper, one teaspoon
- Salt, one teaspoon
- Cauliflower, one head

Instructions

Wash and rinse the cauliflower and let drain well and then pat it dry. Grate the raw cauliflower finely using a hand grater or a food processor. Dump the finely grated cauliflower into a bowl and add the salt, pepper, egg, and onion. Mix all of this together very well. Form the grated cauliflower mixture into pancake shapes and fry them in the melted butter five minutes on each side. If they do not fry long enough, they will break apart when you flip them or remove them from the pan, so do not try to rush them.

Nutrition per serving:

Calories 282, 5 grams net carbs, 26 grams fat, 7 grams protein

5. OATMEAL

Serves one

Ingredients:

- Almond milk, unsweetened, one cup
- Flaxseed, whole, one tablespoon
- Sunflower seeds, one tablespoon
- Chia seeds, one tablespoon
- Salt, one half teaspoon

Instructions

Dump all of the ingredients together into a small pan and bring the mixture to a boil in a saucepan over medium heat. When it comes to a boil, reduce the heat and allow the mix to simmer gently for two to three minutes until the mix is the desired thickness. Drop a pat of butter on the top and enjoy.

Nutrition per serving:

Calories 621, 9 grams net carbs, 62 grams fat, 10 grams protein

6. COCONUT CREAM WITH BERRIES

Serves one

Ingredients:

- Coconut cream, one half cup
- Vanilla extract, one teaspoon
- Strawberries, fresh, two ounces

Instructions

Mix the ingredients together well by using a hand mixer or an immersion mixer if one is available. An added teaspoon of coconut oil will increase the amount of fat in this dish.

Nutrition per serving:

Calories 415, 9 grams net carbs, 42 grams fat, 5 grams protein

7. SEAFOOD OMELET

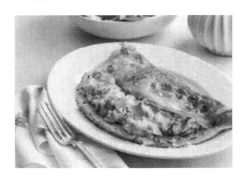

Serves two

Ingredients:

- Shrimp, cooked, five ounces
- Eggs, six
- Butter, two tablespoons
- Olive oil, two tablespoons
- Chives, fresh or dried, one tablespoon
- Mayonnaise, one half cup
- Cumin, ground, one half teaspoon
- Thyme, one quarter teaspoon
- Garlic, two cloves minced
- Red chili pepper, one diced
- Salt, one half teaspoon
- White pepper, one teaspoon

Instructions

Toss the shrimp with the olive oil until it is completely covered and fry it gently with the cumin, garlic, salt, chili pepper, and pepper for five minutes. While the shrimp mix cools beat the eggs and pours them into the skillet. Let the eggs sit undisturbed while they cook until the edges begin to brown and the center has mostly set firm. Then add the chives and the mayonnaise to the shrimp mixture. Pour the shrimp mixture onto the egg that is frying in the skillet and fold the omelet in half, frying for an additional three minutes on each side.

Nutrition per serving:

Calories 872, 4 grams net carbs, 83 grams fat, 27 grams protein

8. SPINACH AND PORK WITH FRIED EGGS

Serves two

Ingredients:

- Spinach, baby, two cups
- Pork loin, smoked, six ounces cut into chunks
- Eggs, four
- Salt, one half teaspoon
- Black pepper, one teaspoon
- Walnuts, chopped, one quarter cup
- Cranberries, one quarter cup frozen
- Butter, three tablespoons

Instructions

Wash, dry, and chop the baby spinach. Fry the spinach in the butter for five minutes stirring continuously. Remove the spinach from the pan and let it drain on a paper towel. Fry the chunks of pork loin in the same skillet for five minutes. Remove the pork from the skillet and then put the cooked baby spinach back in, adding the nuts and cranberries. Stir constantly while this is cooking for five minutes. Pour the mix into a bowl. Fry the eggs and place two on each plate with half of the spinach mixture. Serve with the chunks of fried pork loin.

Nutrition per serving:

Calories 1033, 8 grams net carbs, 99 grams fat, 26 grams protein

9. SMOKED SALMON SANDWICH

Serves two

Ingredients:

<u>TOPPING</u>

- Eggs, four
- Chives, fresh, chop, one tablespoon
- Smoked salmon, three ounces
- Heavy whipping cream, two tablespoons
- Salt, one half teaspoon
- White pepper, one half teaspoon
- Kale, one-ounce chop fine
- Butter, two tablespoons
- Chili powder, one quarter teaspoon
- Olive oil, two tablespoons

<u>SPICY PUMPKIN BREAD</u>

- Lard, one tablespoon
- Pumpkin puree, fourteen ounces
- Coconut oil, .25 cup
- Eggs, three
- Pumpkin seeds, one third cup
- Walnuts, chopped, one third cup
- Baking powder, one tablespoon
- Pumpkin pie spice, two tablespoons
- Flaxseed, one half cup
- Coconut flour, one and one quarter cups

- Almond flour, one and one quarter cups
- Psyllium husk powder, ground, two tablespoons
- Salt, one teaspoon

Instructions

Heat oven to 400. Use the lard to grease a nine by nine pan. Add the baking powder, pumpkin pie spice, nuts, psyllium husk powder, flaxseed, both flours, salt, and seeds into a bowl and mix together well. Use a separate bowl to cream together the oil, pumpkin puree, and egg. Gently pour this mixture into the dry ingredients and fold both together until all of the ingredients are well moistened. Spoon this entire mixture into the greased baking pan and bake it for one hour. Allow the bread to cool completely.

When the bread is done beat together the cream and eggs with the pepper and salt. Scramble the egg mix in the melted butter for five minutes, stirring constantly and then mix in the chili powder. Slice off two slices of the pumpkin bread and place them in the toaster to toast for three minutes. Butter the toasted pumpkin bread and lay each slice on a plate. Top each slice with the kale and the smoked salmon. Place the eggs on top of this and sprinkle with the chives.

Nutrition per serving:

Calories 678, 3 grams net carbs, 55 grams fat, 41 grams protein

10. SHRIMP DEVILED EGGS

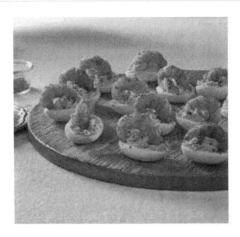

Serves four

Ingredients:

- Chives, chopped, one teaspoon
- Mayonnaise, one quarter cup
- Eggs, four, hard boiled
- Dill sprigs, eight fresh
- Tabasco sauce, one teaspoon
- Shrimp, peeled and deveined, eight large fully cooked*
- Salt, one half teaspoon
- White pepper, one half teaspoon

Instructions

Carefully peel the chilled hard-boiled eggs and then cut them in half the long way and remove the yolks. Put the yolks into a bowl and use a dinner fork to gently mash the yolks and then add the Tabasco, salt, and mayonnaise. Mix all of this together well and then carefully spoon the mixture back into the egg whites. Top each egg with one cooked shrimp and a sprig of dill.

Shrimp are sold whole or peeled and deveined. You can peel them yourself and remove the vein but the cost difference to buy them already peeled and deveined (P & D) in very small and worth the price.

Nutrition per serving:

Calories 163, .5 grams net carbs, 15 grams fat, 7 grams protein

11. SCRAMBLED EGGS WITH HALLOUMI CHEESE

Serves two

Ingredients:

- Eggs, four
- Bacon, four slices
- Salt, one half teaspoon
- Black pepper, one teaspoon
- Chili powder, one quarter teaspoon
- Black olives, pitted if needed, one half cup
- Parsley, fresh, one half cup chop fine
- Scallions, two
- Olive oil, two tablespoons
- Halloumi cheese, diced from a block, three ounces

Instructions

Chop finely the bacon and the cheese. Fry the bacon and the cheese with the scallions in the olive oil for five minutes. While this mixture is frying beat the eggs well with the parsley, pepper, chili powder, and salt. Dump the egg mix onto the bacon cheese mix in the skillet and scramble all together for three minutes while stirring constantly. Add in the olives and cook for three more minutes.

Nutrition per serving:

Calories 667, 4 grams carbs, 59 grams fat, 28 grams protein

12. COCONUT PORRIDGE

Serves one

Ingredients:

- Egg, one
- Salt, one quarter teaspoon
- Coconut oil, one tablespoon
- Coconut cream, four tablespoons
- Psyllium husk powder, ground, one half teaspoon
- Coconut flour, one tablespoon

Instructions

Pour all of the ingredients listed into a pan and mix together well. Cook this mixture over very low heat while stirring constantly until the mixture is the thickness that you desire. Serve the porridge with a spoonful of coconut milk or heavy whipping cream and a few frozen or fresh berries if you like.

Nutrition per serving:

Calories 486, 4 grams net carbs, 49 grams fat, 9 grams protein

13. WESTERN OMELET

Serves two

Ingredients:

- Eggs, six
- Smoked deli ham, five ounces diced small
- Butter, two tablespoons
- Green bell pepper, one-half cup finely chopped
- Yellow onion, one-quarter cup finely chopped
- Shredded sharp cheddar cheese, three ounces
- Sour cream, two tablespoons
- Salt, one half teaspoon
- Black pepper, one teaspoon
- Chives, chopped, one tablespoon
- Thyme, one quarter teaspoon

Instructions

Cream together the eggs and the sour cream together until they are fluffy and season this mix with salt, chives, thyme, and pepper. Sprinkle in just half of the shredded cheese and mix it together well. Cook the peppers, onion, and ham in the melted butter for five minutes while stirring often. Dump the egg mixture carefully over the ham mixture in the skillet and cook for an additional five minutes just sitting still, do not stir. Sprinkle the remainder of the shredded cheese onto the omelet and carefully fold it in half and fry for five more minutes, two and one-half minutes per side.

Nutrition per serving:

Calories 702, 6 grams net carbs, 58 grams fat, 40 grams protein

14. MUSHROOM OMELET

Serves one

Ingredients:

- Eggs, three
- Shredded cheese any style, one ounce
- Mushrooms, one half cup
- Yellow onion, diced fine, one quarter cup
- Salt, one half teaspoon
- White pepper, one quarter teaspoon
- Rosemary, one half teaspoon
- Butter, one tablespoon

Instructions

Break the eggs into a bowl carefully and season them with the pepper, salt, and rosemary. Use a fork or a hand mixer to beat the eggs until they are well mixed and slightly frothy. Pour the egg mixture into the melted butter into the pan. Let the omelet cook over medium heat until the half-inch outer edge has begun to look brown and firm and the center half is still slightly raw and wet. Sprinkle the mushrooms, onions, and cheese onto the omelet, staying mostly near the center and away from the cooked edges. Use a spatula to work the edges free of the omelet off the pan and flip one side over onto the other half. Let the omelet cook five more minutes and remove it from the pan.

Nutrition per omelet:

Calories 510, 4 grams net carbs, 43 grams fat, 25 grams protein

15. FRITTATA WITH FRESH SPINACH

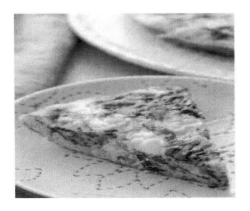

Serves four

Ingredients:

- Eggs, eight
- Heavy whipping cream, one cup
- Salt, one teaspoon
- Black pepper, one teaspoon
- Rosemary, one half teaspoon
- Thyme, one quarter teaspoon
- Shredded sharp cheddar cheese, five ounces
- Spinach, fresh, one cup washed and dried
- Butter, two tablespoons

Instructions

Heat oven to 350. Use one tablespoon of lard to grease a nine by nine-inch baking pan. Use one tablespoon of the butter to fry the bacon in a skillet over medium heat. When the bacon is crispy place the cleaned spinach in the skillet and cooks it until the spinach wilts.

The bacon will break into pieces while you are stirring it with the spinach. During the time the bacon is cooking beat the eggs and the heavy cream together in a small bowl. Pour this mix into the baking pan, then add in the spinach and bacon mix and sprinkle all over the top with the sharp cheddar cheese. Bake for thirty minutes and serve hot.

Nutrition per serving:

Calories 661, 4 grams net carbs, 59 grams fat, 27 grams protein

16. CLASSIC EGGS AND BACON

Serves four

Ingredients:

- Eggs, eight
- Bacon, eight slices
- Parsley, freshly chopped, for garnish
- Cherry tomatoes, one half cup cut in half

Instructions

Fry the bacon in a skillet to desired crispiness and drain it on a paper towel. Leave at least three tablespoons of the leftover bacon grease in the skillet to use to cook the eggs any way you choose—fried or scrambled. When the eggs have almost finished cooking drop the cherry tomatoes into the skillet so that they will be slightly warmed. Serve the eggs with two strips of bacon per person and the warm cherry tomatoes on the side with fresh parsley overall for garnish and taste.

Nutrition per serving:

Calories 272, 1-gram net carbs, 22 grams fat, 15 grams protein

17. PANCAKES WITH BERRIES AND WHIP CREAM

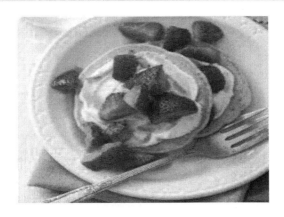

Serves four

Ingredients:

<u>TOPPING</u>

- Heavy whipping cream, one cup cold
- Berries, one cup of strawberries, raspberries, or blackberries

<u>PANCAKE</u>

- Eggs, four
- Butter, two tablespoons
- Psyllium husk powder, ground, one tablespoon
- Cottage cheese, seven ounces

Instructions

Mix the psyllium husk, cottage cheese, and the eggs together well in a small bowl. Let this mix sit for ten minutes so it will thicken.

Use a large skillet to melt the butter completely over medium heat. Use a serving spoon or a ladle to pour pancake batter into the hot butter. Make the pancakes about four inches across. Fry each pancake for four minutes on each side. While the pancakes are cooking place the heavy cream in a bowl and whip with a hand mixer until the cream makes soft peaks. Place the cooked pancakes on a plate and top with the whipped cream and the berries of your choice.

Nutrition per serving:

Calories 425, 5 grams net carbs, 39 grams fat, 13 grams protein

18. MEXICAN SCRAMBLED EGGS

Serves four

Ingredients:

- Eggs, six
- Pickled jalapenos, two chopped fine
- Scallion, one chopped fine
- Butter, two tablespoons
- Shredded cheese, three ounces
- Tomato, one medium chopped fine
- Salt, one half teaspoon
- Black pepper, one teaspoon
- Chili powder, one teaspoon

Instructions

Use a medium-sized skillet over low heat to melt all of the butter and then cook the scallions, jalapenos, and tomatoes for three minutes. Beat the eggs until well mixed and pour them into the pan with the fried vegetables. Scramble the eggs to the desired degree of doneness, adding in the salt, pepper, and chili powder while you stir the eggs. When the eggs are almost done pour in the shredded cheese, stir once, and serve.

Nutrition per serving:

Calories 229, 2 grams net carbs, 18 grams fat, 14 grams protein

19. EGGS WITH AVOCADO

Serves four

Ingredients:

- Eggs, eight
- Avocado, one peeled and cut into eight slices
- Mayonnaise, full fat
- Salt and pepper to taste

Instructions

In a medium-sized pot boil four cups of water. Use a serving spoon to carefully immerse the eggs, one at a time, into the boiling water. Boil the eggs for the time that will give the result desired: eight minutes for hard-boiled, six minutes for medium eggs, and four minutes for soft boiled eggs. Serve the eggs two to a plate with a spoonful of mayonnaise on each plate and two slices of fresh avocado.

Nutrition per serving:

Calories 316, 1-gram net carbs, 29 grams fat, 11 grams protein

20. AVOCADO EGGS WITH BACON

Serves four

Ingredients:

- Eggs, hard-boiled, two
- Avocado, one half
- Salt, one half teaspoon
- Black pepper, one teaspoon
- Thyme, one quarter teaspoon
- Bacon, two ounces
- Olive oil, one teaspoon

Instructions

Heat oven to 350. Use a large spoon to place the eggs carefully into a pan of boiling water and boil them for eight minutes. Immediately place the boiled eggs into a bowl of cold water to make them easier to peel. Carefully peel the boiled eggs and then cut them in half along the length and gently remove the yolks. Put the yolks into a bowl, add the avocado and the oil and mix all these ingredients together well. Add the thyme, pepper, and salt and mix well. Fry the bacon in a skillet until it is crispy or bakes it in the heated oven while you are preparing the eggs. Spoon the egg mix carefully back into the egg white halves and top with bits of crispy crumbled bacon.

Nutrition per serving:

Calories 144, 1-gram net carbs, 13 grams fat, 5 grams protein

21. BUTTERED ASPARAGUS WITH CREAMY EGGS

Serves four

Ingredients:

- Eggs, four
- Butter, five tablespoons divided into two tablespoons and three tablespoons
- Sour cream, one half cup
- Asparagus, twenty-four ounces
- Parmesan cheese, grated, three ounces
- Lemon juice, two tablespoons
- Olive oil, one tablespoon
- Cayenne pepper, one quarter teaspoon
- Salt, one half teaspoon

Instructions

Scramble the eggs in the two tablespoons of butter until they are thoroughly cooked but still slightly wet. Pour the eggs into a blender while they are still hot and add the salt, pepper, parmesan cheese, and sour cream. Blend until this mix is smooth and creamy. Fry the asparagus in a skillet in the olive oil for five minutes. Add in the three tablespoons of butter to the skillet and let it melt completely. Turn off the heat and add in the lemon juice and let the mix set well. After ten minutes return the pan to the heat, add in the asparagus, and stir to mix completely. Place all items on a plate and serve.

Nutrition per serving:

Calories 527, 6 grams net carbs, 48 grams fat, 18 grams protein

22. NO BREAD BREAKFAST SANDWICH

Serves four

Ingredients:

- Eggs, four
- Smoked deli ham, two ounces
- Cheddar cheese, two thick slices from a block, about one-half-inch thick
- Tabasco sauce, one half teaspoon
- Salt, one half teaspoon
- Black pepper, one teaspoon
- Butter, two tablespoons

Instructions

Fry the eggs to over medium in the melted butter and then sprinkle them with salt and pepper. Place one fried egg on each of four plates for serving, one on each plate Top each egg with one slice of cheese and half of the ham. Drizzle each stack with tabasco sauce.

Nutrition per serving:

Calories 354, 2 grams net carbs, 30 grams fat, 20 grams protein

23. MUSHROOM AND CHEESE FRITTATA

Serves four

Ingredients:

<u>VINAIGRETTE</u>

- Olive oil, four tablespoons
- White wine vinegar, one tablespoon
- Black pepper, ground, one teaspoon
- Salt, one half teaspoon

<u>FRITTATA</u>

- Mushrooms, button, one cup
- Parsley, chopped from fresh, one tablespoon
- Scallions, six diced
- Kale, rinsed and dried, two cups
- Mayonnaise, one cup
- Butter, three tablespoons
- Shredded cheese, one cup
- Eggs, ten
- Black pepper, ground, one teaspoon
- Salt, one half teaspoon

Instructions

Heat oven to 350. Pour all of the vinaigrette ingredients into a jar with a lid. Shake this very well and set it aside. Fry the mushrooms, parsley, and scallions with the pepper and salt added for five minutes in the melted butter. In a different bowl mix together well the mayonnaise, cheese, and eggs. Add the scallion, mushroom, and parsley mix to the egg mix and pour all of it into a greased eight by eight-inch baking dish. Bake the frittata for forty minutes. Serve with drizzles of the vinaigrette.

Nutrition per serving:

Calories 1061, 6 grams net carbs, 101 grams fat, 32 grams protein

24. EGG MUFFINS

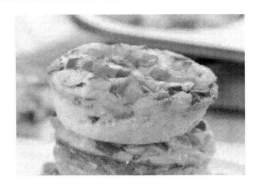

Serves six

Ingredients:

- Eggs, twelve
- Bacon, cooked, six slices
- Scallions, two, chopped finely
- Salt, one teaspoon
- Pepper, one teaspoon
- Pesto, red or green, two tablespoons
- Rosemary, one teaspoon
- Thyme, one quarter teaspoon
- Shredded cheddar cheese, one half cup
- Shredded mozzarella cheese, one half cup

Instructions

Heat oven to 350. Set paper or foil baking cups in all twelve cups of a twelve-cup muffin pan. Chop the scallions and the bacon and put a little bit in each cup. Beat the eggs with the cheese, thyme, rosemary, pesto, salt, and pepper. Divide the egg mixture into the baking cups. Bake them for twenty minutes.

Nutrition per serving:

Calories 336, 2 grams net carbs, 26 grams fat, 23 grams protein

25. CHIA PUDDING

Serves one

Ingredients:

- Cinnamon, one tablespoon
- Coconut milk, one cup
- Vanilla extract, one teaspoon
- Chia seeds, two tablespoons

Instructions

Place all of the ingredients into a glass jar or bowl. Mix together and cover well and place in the refrigerator overnight or for at least four hours. The pudding will thicken during that time, and the chia seeds will have gelled, making this a smooth, creamy breakfast pudding.

Nutrition per serving:

Calories 461, 7 grams net carbs, 44 grams fat, 7 grams protein

26. SALMON FILLED AVOCADO

Serves two

Ingredients:

- Avocados, two
- Lemon juice, two tablespoons
- Salt, one half teaspoon
- Black pepper, one teaspoon
- Sour cream, one cup
- Smoked salmon, six ounces

Instructions

Gently peel the raw avocados and cut them in half the long way and then remove the pit. Spoon the sour cream into the holes where the pit was and place the smoked salmon on top of the sour cream. Drizzle on the lemon juice and then season to taste with the salt and the pepper.

Nutrition per serving:

Calories 911, 6 grams net carbs, 71 grams fat, 58 grams protein

27. RUTABAGA FRITTERS WITH AVOCADO

Serves four

Ingredients:

MAYONNAISE DRESSING

- Ranch seasoning, one tablespoon
- Mayonnaise, one cup

FRITTERS

- Eggs, four
- Butter, for frying, four tablespoons
- Rutabaga, fifteen ounces
- Pepper, one half teaspoon
- Salt, one half teaspoon
- Halloumi cheese, eight ounces
- Turmeric, one quarter teaspoon
- Coconut flour, three tablespoons

Serve with avocado slices and leafy greens of your choice

Instructions

Heat oven to 250. Rinse the rutabaga well and peel it. Grate the rutabaga finely using a food processor or a hand grater. Use the same process for shredding the cheese. Use a large bowl to mix the coconut flour with the grated rutabaga, pepper, salt, cheese, turmeric, and eggs and let this mixture stand for ten minutes. Form the mixture into twelve equal-sized patties and fry them, three or four at a time, in the melted butter over medium heat. Fry the patties for five minutes on each side. Put the already cooked patties in the oven to keep them warm while you are cooking the rest. Top with the ranch dressing to serve.

Nutrition per serving:

Calories 1211, 14 grams net carbs, 113 grams fat, 25 grams protein

28. BACON MUSHROOM BREAKFAST CASSEROLE

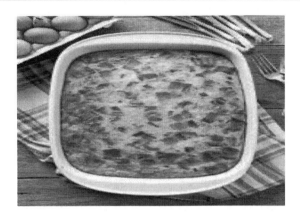

Serves four

Ingredients:

- Eggs, eight
- Bacon, twelve ounces
- Heavy whipping cream, one cup
- Butter, two tablespoons
- Salt, one teaspoon
- Pepper, one teaspoon
- Cheddar cheese, shredded, five ounces
- Mushrooms, six ounces

Instructions

Heat oven to 400. Rinse and dry the mushrooms and chop them. Chop the bacon into bite-size pieces. Fry the bacon bits and the mushrooms in the butter for five minutes over medium heat. Use one tablespoon of lard to grease a nine by thirteen-inch baking dish and add the mushroom and bacon mixture to it. Beat the cream with the eggs, cheese, pepper, and salt in a bowl and pour into the baking dish on top of the bacon and mushrooms. Bake this for forty minutes.

Nutrition per serving:

Calories 876, 6 grams net carbs, 81 grams fat, 31 grams protein

29. BAKED EGGS

Serves one

Ingredients:

- Eggs, two
- Ground pork, three ounces cooked
- Shredded cheddar cheese, two ounces

Instructions

Heat oven to 400. Use one tablespoon of lard to grease a small baking pan about a five by five-inch. Lay the cooked ground pork in the pan. Then crack both eggs and over the top of the cooked pork. Sprinkle all over the top with shredded cheese and bake for fifteen minutes.

Nutrition per serving:

Calories 509, 2 grams net carbs, 36 grams fat, 42 grams protein

30. KETO BLUEBERRY MUFFINS

Serves six to twelve

Ingredients:

- Lemon zest, one tablespoon
- Blueberries, fresh, one half cup
- Vanilla, one teaspoon
- Eggs, three large
- Almond milk, unsweetened
- Butter, one-third cup melted
- Salt, one half teaspoon
- Baking soda, one half teaspoon
- Baking powder, one and one half teaspoon
- Almond flour, two and one half cups

Instructions

Heat oven to 350. Use paper or foil liners to line all twelve cups of a twelve cup muffin pan. Use a large bowl to mix the almond flour with the salt, baking soda, and baking powder. Then mix in the vanilla, eggs, almond milk, and melted butter just until the dry ingredients are wet. Then gently fold in the lemon zest and the blueberries until they are mixed evenly into the batter. Divide the batter among the twelve cups until all of the batter is used. Bake the muffins twenty to twenty-five minutes until a knife inserted in the center of one comes out clean. Let them cool slightly before eating.

Nutrition per muffin:

Calories 229, 4 grams net carbs, 19 grams fat, 8 grams protein

31. TACO BREAKFAST SKILLET

Serves six

Ingredients:

- Cilantro, two tablespoons fresh torn
- Jalapeno, one sliced
- Salsa, one quarter cup
- Green onions, two sliced thin
- Black olives, one quarter cup sliced
- Avocado, one medium peeled, pitted, cubed
- Roma tomato, one diced
- Heavy cream, one quarter cup
- Sharp cheddar cheese, shredded, one and one-half cup divided
- Eggs, ten
- Water, two-thirds cup
- Taco seasoning, four tablespoons
- Ground beef, one pound

Instructions

Heat oven to 375. Cook the ground beef until fully cooked in a large skillet over medium heat. Drain off the excess fat. Add the taco seasoning and the water to the meat back in the skillet. Turn the heat down to low and let the mix simmer until the water has almost disappeared and the seasoning is coating the meat, for about five minutes. Beat the eggs together well in a large bowl and add the heavy cream and one cup of the cheese and mix well. Pour the meat mixture into a greased nine by nine baking dish and pour the egg mixture on top. Bake this for thirty minutes. Cover the mix with the rest of the shredded cheese, green onion, olives, tomato, and avocado. Serve with the cilantro, jalapeno, salsa, and sour cream on the side for garnish.

Nutrition per serving:

Calories 563, 9 grams carbs, 44 grams fat, 32 grams protein

32. CREAM CHEESE PANCAKES

Serves one

Ingredients:

- Cinnamon, one teaspoon
- Eggs, two
- Cream cheese, two ounces
- Butter, two tablespoons

Instructions

Make a smooth batter by mixing well all of the ingredients. Let the batter rest for five minutes. Pour in one-quarter of the batter into melted butter in a skillet over medium heat. Cook all of the pancakes for about two to three minutes on each side. Serve them with fruit if desired.

Nutrition info:

Calories 344, 3 grams net carbs, 29 grams fat, 17 grams protein

33. KETO CLOUD BREAD

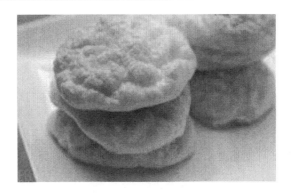

This recipe is perfect for any meal. Have it for breakfast with a bit of keto strawberry jam as an occasional treat. And look for the strawberry jam recipe in this book.

Ingredients:

- Salt, one quarter teaspoon
- Cream of tartar, one quarter teaspoon
- Cream cheese, three tablespoons at room temperature
- Eggs, three at room temperature

Instructions

Heat oven to 350. Cover two cookie sheets with parchment paper. Separate the three eggs and put the whites in one bowl and the yolks in another. Blend the cream cheese into the egg yolks. Add cream of tartar and salt to the egg whites and beat them with a hand mixer or stand mixer until they form stiff peaks. Slowly fold the yolk mixture into the egg white mixture using a spatula; mix until there are no yellow streaks remaining. Spoon the mixture onto the parchment paper covered cookie sheets in mounds about three inches across and one half inch high. Bake for thirty minutes on the middle oven rack. Allow the bread to cool completely before using.

Nutrition per piece:

Calories 35, .4 grams carbs, 2.8-gram fat, 2.2 grams protein

Chapter Eight

KETO LUNCH AND DINNER RECIPES

These recipes will work for either lunch menus or dinner menus. A simple keto style meal for lunch or dinner would be a protein choice – meat, poultry, or fish – with a low carb vegetable choice or a leafy salad. But sometimes you want to make something creative or show off an impressive dish for a dinner party. These recipes will delight family and friends alike.

1. TUNA CASSEROLE

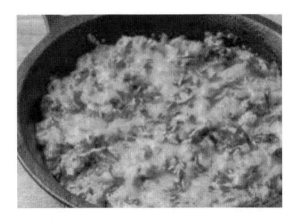

Serves four

Ingredients:

- Tuna in oil, sixteen ounces, drained
- Butter, two tablespoons
- Salt, one half teaspoon
- Black pepper, one teaspoon
- Chili powder, one teaspoon
- Celery, six stalks
- Green bell pepper, one
- Yellow onion, one
- Parmesan cheese, grated, four ounces
- Mayonnaise, one cup

Instructions

Heat the oven to 400. Chop the onion, bell pepper, and celery very fine and fry in the melted butter for five minutes. Stir together with the chili powder, parmesan cheese, tuna, and mayonnaise. Use lard to grease an eight by eight-inch or nine by a nine-inch baking pan.

Add the tuna mixture into the fried vegetables and spoon the mix into the baking pan. Bake it for twenty minutes.

Nutrition per serving:

Calories 953, 5 grams net carbs, 83 grams fat, 43 grams protein

2. WHITE FISH WITH CURRY AND COCONUT

Serves four

Ingredients:

- Whitefish or salmon, twenty-five ounces approximately in four pieces
- Salt, one teaspoon
- Pepper, one teaspoon
- Broccoli or cauliflower, two cups
- Cilantro, fresh, chopped, one half cup
- Coconut cream, fourteen ounces
- Curry paste, green or red, two tablespoons
- Butter or ghee, four tablespoons
- Lard to grease baking pan

Instructions

Heat the oven to 400. Use two tablespoons of lard to grease a nine by thirteen-inch baking pan and lay the fish pieces in it. Salt and pepper the fish pieces and lay a pat of butter on top of each slice. Blend the coconut cream, curry paste, and chopped cilantro in a bowl until smooth and then spoon this mix over the fish. Bake the fish for twenty minutes. While the fish is baking cut the cauliflower or the broccoli into bite-size florets and then boil them in salt water for five minutes.

Nutrition per serving:

Calories 880, 9 grams net carbs, 75 grams fat, 42 grams protein

3. CREAMY FISH CASSEROLE

Serves four

Ingredients:

- Whitefish, twenty-five ounces approximately, cut into four serving pieces
- Capers, small, two tablespoons
- Scallions, six
- Broccoli, sixteen ounces
- Butter, three tablespoons
- Dijon mustard, one tablespoon
- Heavy whipping cream, one and one quarter cups
- Parsley, dried, one tablespoon
- Black pepper, one teaspoon
- Salt, one teaspoon
- Olive oil, two tablespoons

Instructions

Heat the oven to 400. Rinse and dry the broccoli and cut it into florets leaving stems on. Use the oil to fry the broccoli for five minutes stirring occasionally. Add in the scallions and the capers. Fry for three minutes, stirring once. Use butter to grease a nine by thirteen-inch baking dish. Place the veggies in the baking dish. Lay the fish in on top of the veggies. In a small bowl mix the parsley, whipping cream, and the mustard and pour this mix on top of the vegetables and fish in the baking pan. Bake for thirty minutes. Lay six pats of butter on top in random places and let it melt before serving. Serve with a bowl of leafy greens.

Nutrition per serving:

Calories 822, 8 grams net carbs, 69 grams fat, 41 grams protein

4. SPINACH AND GOAT CHEESE PIE

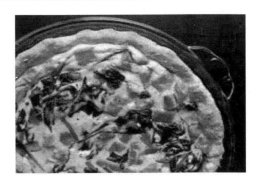

Serves six

Ingredients:

- EGG BATTER
- Sour cream, one cup
- Eggs, five
- Salt, one half teaspoon
- Black pepper, one teaspoon

<u>PIE CRUST</u>

- Almond flour, one and one half cups
- Butter, two tablespoons
- Salt, one half teaspoon
- Egg, one
- Psyllium husk powder, ground, one tablespoon
- Sesame seeds

GOAT CHEESE AND SPINACH FILLING

- Spinach, fresh, eight ounces
- Goat cheese, six ounces sliced
- Salt, one half teaspoon
- Black pepper, one teaspoon
- Cheddar cheese, shredded, one half cup
- Nutmeg, ground, one half teaspoon
- Garlic, one clove
- Butter, two tablespoons

Instructions

Heat the oven to 350. Use a fork to mix the ingredients for the dough until you make a ball of dough. Press this dough into a greased springform pan covering the bottom and the sides. Use a fork to poke holes randomly in the crust, about ten to fifteen sets. Bake the empty pie shell for ten minutes. Cream together the eggs, sour cream, salt, and pepper. Chop the garlic and the spinach fine. Fry the garlic and the spinach in the hot butter for five minutes stirring occasionally. Put this mix into the pie shell and sprinkle the grated cheese over the top. Pour the creamed egg mixture over all ingredients and place the goat cheese on top. Bake for forty-five minutes.

Nutrition per serving:

Calories 643, 4 grams net carbs, 58 grams fat, 24 grams protein

5. AVOCADO PIE

Serves four

Ingredients:

PIE CRUST

- Coconut flour, four tablespoons
- Almond flour, three-fourths of a cup
- Psyllium husk powder, ground, one tablespoon
- Sesame seeds, four tablespoons
- Water, four tablespoons
- Egg, one
- Olive oil, three tablespoons
- Salt, one quarter teaspoon
- Baking powder, one teaspoon

FILLING

- Eggs, three
- Mayonnaise, one cup
- Shredded cheese, one and one quarter cups
- Onion powder, one teaspoon
- Red chili pepper, one chop fine
- Cilantro, fresh chopped, two tablespoons
- Cream cheese, one half cup
- Salt, one half teaspoon
- Avocados, two ripe

Instructions

Heat the oven to 350. Use a fork to mix the crust ingredients in a bowl or use a food processor to mix them. Use two tablespoons of lard to grease a deep pie pan. Lay the dough ball into the pie dish, using your fingers or a spatula to spread it all over the bottom of the pan and up the sides. Poke ten to fifteen sets of holes in the bottom with a dinner fork and bake the crust empty for ten minutes. Wash and peel the avocado and remove the pit, then dice the avocado. Clean the seeds out of the chili and dice it. Mix together the diced chili and the diced avocado with the rest of the ingredients. Spoon this mix into the pre-baked crust and bake all for an additional forty minutes.

Nutrition per serving:

Calories 1146, 9 grams net carbs, 109 grams fat, 26 grams protein

6. TEX MEX STUFFED ZUCCHINI BOATS

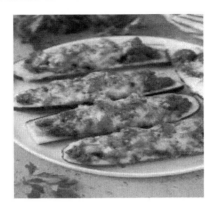

Serves four

Ingredients:

- Ground beef, one pound
- Zucchini, two medium-sized
- Cilantro, fresh, chopped fine, one half cup
- Cheddar cheese, shredded, one and one half cups
- Olive oil, one tablespoon
- Salt, one teaspoon
- Tex Mex seasoning, two tablespoons
- Olive oil or butter, two tablespoons

Instructions

Heat the oven to 400. Cut both zucchinis in half down the length and remove the seeds but do not peel. Cook the ground beef in the olive oil until it is brown, about ten minutes. Stir in the salt and the Tex Mex seasoning and let this cook until all of the liquid has cooked away. Use two tablespoons of lard to grease a nine by thirteen-inch baking pan and lay the zucchini halves in it cut side up. Stir one-third of the shredded cheese into the meat mixture and add the cilantro. Fill the halves of the zucchini evenly with the meat and cheese mix. Use the rest of the shredded cheese to sprinkle on the top. Bake the zucchini boats for twenty minutes.

Nutrition per serving:

Calories 601, 6 grams net carbs, 49 grams fat, 33 grams protein

7. BRUSSEL SPROUTS AND HAMBURGER GRATIN

Serves four

Ingredients:

- Ground beef, one pound
- Bacon, eight ounces, diced small
- Brussel sprouts, fifteen ounces, cut in half
- Salt, one teaspoon
- Black pepper, one teaspoon
- Thyme, one half teaspoon
- Cheddar cheese, shredded, one cup
- Italian seasoning, one tablespoon
- Sour cream, four tablespoons
- Butter, two tablespoons

Instructions

Heat the oven to 425. Fry bacon and Brussel sprouts in butter for five minutes. Stir in the sour cream and pour this mix into a greased eight by eight-inch baking pan. Cook the ground beef and season with the salt and pepper, then add this mix to the baking pan. Top with the herbs and the shredded cheese. Bake for twenty minutes.

Nutrition per serving:

Calories 770, 8 grams net carbs, 62 grams fat, 42 grams protein

8. ITALIAN CABBAGE STIR FRY

Serves four

Ingredients:

- Ground beef, twenty ounces
- Green cabbage, twenty-five ounces
- Tomato paste, one tablespoon
- White wine vinegar, one tablespoon
- Pepper, one teaspoon
- Salt, one teaspoon
- Onion powder, one teaspoon
- Sour cream, one cup for serving
- Basil, fresh, one half cup
- Leeks, three, slice thin
- Garlic, two cloves, chopped fine
- Rosemary, one teaspoon
- Butter, six tablespoons

Instructions

Rinse and dry the green cabbage and shred it finely. Use three tablespoons of the butter to fry the shredded cabbage for ten minutes, stirring frequently. Stir in the salt, pepper, vinegar, and onion powder and mix this well, and then remove the cabbage mix to a bowl. Place the rest of the butter into the skillet and add in the garlic and the leeks and cook these for three minutes. Pour in the meat and cook for ten more minutes, stirring often. Mix in the tomato paste and the reserved cabbage and stir well.

Nutrition per serving:

Calories 1003, 9 grams net carbs, 91 grams fat, 33 grams protein

9. TEX MEX CASSEROLE

Serves four

Ingredients:

TO SERVE

- Sour cream, one cup
- Scallion, one chopped fine
- Guacamole, one cup
- Leafy greens, one cup

CASSEROLE

- Ground beef, two pounds
- Tex Mex seasoning, three tablespoons
- Monterey Jack cheese, shredded, one cup
- Jalapenos, pickled, two ounces
- Tomatoes, crushed, seven ounces (canned is fine)
- Butter, two ounces

Instructions

Heat the oven to 400. Cook the ground beef completely in the melted butter. Add in the Tex Mex seasoning and the tomatoes and mix well. Use two tablespoons lard to grease an eight by eight-inch baking pan and put the meat mixture in it. Scatter the cheese and the jalapenos on top of the meat and bake all for twenty-five minutes. While the meat mix is baking chop up the scallion very fine and mix it with the sour cream. Serve the meat mix with a spoon of the sour cream, a spoon of guacamole, and some of the leafy greens on the side.

Nutrition per serving:

Calories 860, 8 grams net carbs, 69 grams fat, 49 grams protein

10. HERBED GRILLED CHICKEN

Serves four

Ingredients:

- Chicken thighs, eight boneless
- Dried fennel seeds, one teaspoon
- Peppercorns, whole, one teaspoon
- Garlic, minced, two teaspoons
- Thyme, dried, one tablespoon
- Rosemary, dried, one tablespoon
- Salt, one half teaspoon
- Black pepper, one teaspoon

Instructions

Mix together all of the spices with the salt and pepper in a small bowl. Press the chicken thighs into the seasoning bowl on both sides. Cover the thighs on a plate and place them in the refrigerator for two hours. Grill the thighs on a grill or cook under the broiler for eight minutes on each side. Serve with a low carb vegetable or fresh greens.

Nutrition per piece:

Calories 275, 1 gram net carbs, 17 grams fat, 1 gram protein

11. HAM CHEESE AND CHIVE SOUFFLÉ

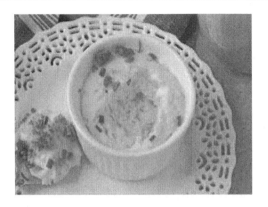

Serves four

Ingredients:

- Ham, diced, six ounces
- Cheddar cheese, shredded, one cup
- Yellow onion, one small peeled and diced
- Heavy cream, one half cup
- Eggs, six large
- Chives, chopped fresh, two tablespoons
- Salt, one teaspoon
- Black pepper, one teaspoon
- Garlic, minced, two tablespoons
- Olive oil, two tablespoons

Instructions

Heat the oven to 400. Use one tablespoon of lard to grease four six-ounce ramekins or another oven-safe dish. Fry the onion and the garlic in the olive oil for five minutes. Mix all of the remaining ingredients together in a bowl, then add the fried onions and garlic to the bowl and mix well. Divide the mix among the oven dishes and cook them for twenty-five minutes.

Nutrition per serving:

Calories 460, 5 grams net carbs, 38 grams fat, 24 grams protein

12. DEVILED EGG SALAD

Serves six

Ingredients:

- Eggs, twelve larges
- Salt, one teaspoon
- Black pepper, one teaspoon
- Green onion, two sliced thinly
- Crushed red pepper flakes, one tablespoon (optional)
- Celery, one stalk diced
- Paprika, one half teaspoon
- Apple cider vinegar
- Dijon mustard, two tablespoons
- Mayonnaise, six tablespoons

Instructions

Cook the eggs to hard-boiled by placing them in a pot of cold water, bringing the water to a boil, then boiling for ten minutes. Immediately put the pot in the sink and run cold water in it until the eggs are cooled to the touch. When the eggs have cooled completely then peel them and chop them into bite-sized chunks. In a large bowl mix together the paprika, salt, pepper, vinegar, mustard, and mayonnaise until creamy. Add in the crushed pepper (optional), celery, green onion, and the egg chunks. Keep the salad well chilled until time to serve it. Serve on a bed of leafy greens.

Nutrition per serving:

Calories 245, 1-gram net carbs, 20 grams fat, 13 grams protein

13. FAJITA CHICKEN CASSEROLE

Serves four

Ingredients:

- Chicken, fully cooked, three cups
- Yellow onion, one
- Red bell pepper, one
- Black pepper, one teaspoon
- Salt, one teaspoon
- Cheddar cheese, shredded, seven ounces or Mexican blend
- Mayonnaise, one half cup
- Cream cheese, eight ounces, softened to room temperature
- Taco seasoning, two tablespoons

Instructions

Heat the oven to 400. Peel the onion and clean the bell pepper and chop both into chunks. Keep one-third of the shredded cheese off to the side. Mix together the onion, bell pepper, mayonnaise, taco seasoning, salt, pepper, cream cheese, chicken, and the remainder of the shredded cheese. Place all of this mix into a greased eight by eight-inch or nine by nine-inch baking pan and sprinkle the reserved cheese over the top. Bake for twenty minutes.

Nutrition per serving:

Calories 1148, 10 grams net carbs, 98 grams fat, 57 grams protein

14. GARAM CHICKEN MASALA

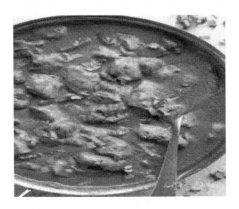

Serves four

Ingredients:

CHICKEN

- Chicken breast, diced into bite-size pieces, three cups

- Parsley, fresh, chopped fine, one tablespoon

- Red bell pepper, one fine diced

- Salt, one teaspoon

- Heavy whipping cream or coconut cream, one- and one-half cups

- Butter or ghee, three tablespoons

GARAM MASALA

- Cumin, ground, one teaspoon
- Cardamom, ground, one teaspoon
- Nutmeg, ground, one half teaspoon

143

- Chili powder, one teaspoon
- Ginger, ground, one teaspoon
- Turmeric, ground, one teaspoon
- Paprika, powder, one teaspoon

Instructions

Heat the oven to 400. Mix all of the Garam Masala spices together in a bowl. Fry the chicken in the melted butter over medium heat for ten minutes. Sprinkle half of the Garam Masala onto the chicken while it is cooking and mix well. Place all of the cooked chicken mixtures into a well-greased nine by thirteen-inch baking dish, including the juice in the skillet. Stir the finely diced bell pepper in with the rest of the masala mix and the coconut cream. Top the chicken in the baking dish with this mixture. Bake for thirty minutes. Sprinkle the parsley over the cooked chicken.

Nutrition per serving:

Calories 628, 6 grams net carbs, 51 grams fat, 38 grams protein

15. CHICKEN CABBAGE AND ONIONS

Serves two

Ingredients:

- Rotisserie chicken or cooked chicken breast, two cups
- Red onion, one half of medium onion
- Green cabbage, one cup finely shredded
- Pepper, one teaspoon
- Salt, one teaspoon
- Greek yogurt, one half cup
- Olive oil, one tablespoon

Instructions

Lay rounds of the shredded cabbage on two dinner plates and top these with thin slices of the red onions. Pour the olive oil over the onions and cabbage in thin lines and season with the salt and pepper. Place spoons of Greek yogurt besides the vegetable mix and top the onions and cabbage with the diced cooked chicken.

Nutrition per serving:

Calories 1041, 7 grams net carbs, 91 grams fat, 48 grams protein

16. CHICKEN LEGS WITH COLESLAW

Serves four

Ingredients:

<u>CHICKEN</u>

- Chicken legs, two pounds
- Olive oil, two tablespoons
- Sour cream, one half cup
- Coconut, shredded, unsweetened, three ounces
- Pork rinds, six ounces
- Olive oil, four tablespoons
- Salt, one teaspoon
- Jerk seasoning, two tablespoons

<u>COLESLAW</u>

- Mayonnaise, one cup
- Pepper, one teaspoon
- Salt, one half teaspoon
- Green cabbage, two cups chopped finely

Instructions

Heat the oven to 350. Mix in a bowl the sour cream with the salt and the jerk seasoning. Pour this over the chicken legs in a bowl and let them marinate for thirty minutes. Throw away the marinade. Crush the pork rinds and mix in the coconut. Roll the chicken legs in the coconut pork rind mixture. Lay the chicken legs on an oven rack that is over a baking dish or cookie sheet. Bake the chicken for forty-five minutes, turning it over after twenty minutes. During the time that the chicken is baking, you can make the coleslaw by coarsely shredding or chopping the cabbage and mixing it well with the rest of the ingredients. Serve the chicken with the slaw.

Nutrition per serving:

Calories 1370, 7 grams net carbs, 116 grams fat, 68 grams protein

17. RUTABAGA AND PAPRIKA CHICKEN

Serves four

Ingredients:

- Chicken thighs, eight boneless
- Rutabaga, one large
- Salt, one teaspoon
- Pepper one teaspoon
- Mayonnaise, one cup
- Paprika, one tablespoon
- Olive oil, four tablespoons

Instructions

Heat the oven to 400. Use two tablespoons of lard to grease a nine by thirteen-inch baking dish and lay the chicken pieces in it. Wash and dry the outside of the rutabaga and then peel it and cut it into two-inch long pieces. Add the rutabaga to the chicken in the baking dish and season both ingredients with the salt, pepper, and paprika. Pour the olive oil over the top of all the ingredients and bake for forty-five minutes uncovered. Serve with the mayonnaise on the side.

Nutrition per serving:

Calories 1165, 15 grams net carbs, 103 grams fat, 40 grams protein

18. CHICKEN BACON RANCH CASSEROLE

Serves eight

Ingredients:

- Chicken thighs, cooked and diced, two pounds
- Bacon, cooked, four slices
- Cheddar cheese, two cups shredded and divided
- Yellow onion, diced, one quarter cup
- Sour cream, one half cup
- Mayonnaise, one cup
- Cream cheese, eight ounces room temperature
- Broccoli, one pound chopped small and steamed
- Garlic powder, two teaspoons
- Parsley, chopped, one tablespoon
- Salt, one teaspoon
- Black pepper, one teaspoon

Instructions

Heat the oven to 350. Use two tablespoons of lard to grease a thirteen by nine-inch baking dish. Cream together the sour cream, mayonnaise, and cream cheese and stir in the pepper, salt, garlic powder, and parsley. Mix in the broccoli, onion, chicken, bacon, and one and one-half cups of the cheese. Put this mix into the baking pan and sprinkle the rest of the cheese over the top of the casserole and bake for thirty minutes.

Nutrition per serving:

Calories 545, 5 grams net carbs, 42 grams fat, 38 grams protein

19. PIMIENTO CHEESE MEATBALLS

Serves four

Ingredients:

MEATBALLS

- Ground beef, two pounds
- Salt, one teaspoon
- Pepper, one teaspoon
- Butter, two tablespoons for frying
- Egg, one

PIMIENTO CHEESE

- Pimientos, one quarter cup
- Mayonnaise, one half cup
- Cheddar cheese, grated, one half cup
- Cayenne pepper, one quarter teaspoon
- Dijon mustard, one tablespoon
- Paprika powder or chili powder, one teaspoon

Instructions

Put all of the ingredients for the pimiento cheese in a bowl and mix it together and let this mix sit for five minutes. Then add in the salt, pepper, egg, and ground beef and mix well with your hands or a spoon. Form the mix into golf ball-sized meatballs and fry the meatballs in the melted butter for ten minutes on each side. Serve with a salad of leafy greens on the side.

Nutrition per serving:

Calories 660, 1 gram net carbs, 53 grams fat, 42 grams protein

20. SLOPPY JOES

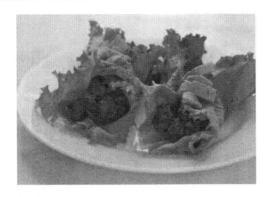

Serves four

Ingredients:

- Ground beef, one pound
- Salt, one teaspoon
- Black pepper, one teaspoon
- Worcestershire sauce, two teaspoons
- Tomato paste, one quarter cup
- Beef broth, three quarters cup
- Garlic, minced, two tablespoons
- Yellow onion, one small diced finely
- Celery, one stalk diced finely

Instructions

Cook the beef in a skillet over medium heat until it is well browned using a spatula or a spoon to break it up into small fine pieces. When the meat is thoroughly browned add in the garlic, onion, and celery and cook for five more minutes. Blend in the leftover ingredients and mix together well. Turn down the heat and let the mix simmer for twenty minutes until it begins to thicken. Serve the sloppy joes on keto cloud bread or on leaf lettuce.

Nutrition per serving:

Calories 240, 4.5 grams net carbs, 7.5 grams fat, 36 grams protein

21. PIGS IN A BLANKET

Serves six

Ingredients:

- Hot dogs, all-beef, twelve
- Mozzarella cheese, shredded, two cups
- Sesame seeds, one teaspoon
- Eggs, two whisked
- Coconut flour, one half cup
- Cream cheese, two ounces at room temperature
- Baking powder, one half teaspoon
- Oregano, dried, one teaspoon
- Garlic powder, one half teaspoon
- Onion powder, one teaspoon

Instructions

Heat oven to 400. Lay parchment paper on a cookie sheet. Put the cream cheese and mozzarella in a heatproof bowl and microwave for three minutes, then mix it together well until creamy. In another bowl mix together the eggs, baking powder, garlic powder, onion powder, oregano, and coconut flour until they are well mixed. Mix in the melted cheese. Wet your hands before sticking them in the dough because it will be sticky. Separate the dough into twelve equal-sized pieces and roll them into balls. Roll the balls of dough out into circles the same width as the hot dog is long. Roll up each hotdog with a circle of dough and lay them on the parchment paper on the cookie sheet. Sprinkle the sesame seeds on the dough and then bake for fifteen to twenty minutes until they are browned.

Nutrition per two hot dogs:

Calories 370, 7.5 grams net carbs, 23.5 grams fat, 24.5 grams protein

22. BAKED FISH STICKS

Serves four

Ingredients:

- Cod fillets, fresh, twelve ounces
- Egg, one large
- Pork rinds, one three and one half ounce bag
- Coconut flour, one and one half tablespoons

Instructions

Heat the oven to 400. Cut the codfish into strips and season them with the salt and pepper. Evenly coat the fish strips with the coconut flour. Smash the pork rinds into fine crumbs. Beat the water and egg white together well and use it to dip the fish strips into, and then into the pork rinds. Gently lay the fish sticks on a well-greased cookie sheet and bake them for fifteen minutes.

Nutrition per serving:

Calories 270, 1 gram net carbs, 11.5 grams fat, 38 grams protein

23. LEMON PARMESAN BAKED COD

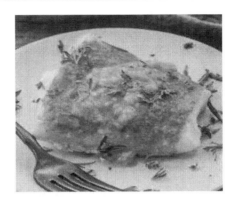

Serves four

Ingredients:

- Cod fillets, boneless, two pounds
- Lemon zest, one tablespoon
- Parsley, chopped, one tablespoon
- Paprika, one teaspoon
- Parmesan cheese, grated, three-fourths cup
- Garlic, minced, two tablespoons
- Butter, melted, one quarter cup

Instructions

Heat the oven to 400. Lay parchment paper over a cookie sheet. Cream together the garlic and butter in one bowl and mix the paprika with the parmesan in another bowl. Dip the fillets in the butter on both sides one by one and then roll them in the parmesan mixture. Lay the fillets on the cookie sheet. When all of the fillets are on the cookie sheet sprinkle them with the lemon zest and the parsley and bake for twenty minutes until the flesh of the fish separates easily with a fork.

Nutrition per serving:

Calories 320, 1 gram net carbs, 17.5 grams fat, 36.5 grams protein

24. BACON-WRAPPED MEATLOAF

Serves four

Ingredients:

- Ground beef, two pounds
- Egg, one
- Cheddar cheese, shredded, one half cup
- Heavy cream, for the gravy
- Bacon, seven slices
- Soy sauce, one tablespoon
- Black pepper, one teaspoon
- Salt, one teaspoon
- Basil, dried one teaspoon
- Oregano, dried, one teaspoon
- Mayonnaise, one half cup
- Yellow onion, one, chopped fine
- Butter, two tablespoons

Instructions

Heat the oven to 400. In the melted butter fry the onion for five minutes. Put the meat into a large bowl. Mix in the butter and onion mixture along with the remainder of the ingredients except for the bacon and the heavy cream. Use your hands to mix this together well, but do not overwork the mixture because this will make the meatloaf too dry. Use two tablespoons of lard to grease a nine-inch loaf dish. Make the meat mixture into a loaf shape and wrap the bacon around it. Bake for one hour. Remove the meat from the baking pan and pour the juices into a bowl with the whipping cream and mix well. Top the individual slices with the cream gravy mixture.

Nutrition per serving:

Calories 1038, 6 grams net carbs, 90 grams fat, 48 grams protein

25. ASIAN MEATBALLS WITH BASIL SAUCE

Serves four

Ingredients:

ASIAN MEATBALLS

- Ground pork, two pounds
- Black pepper, one teaspoon
- Ginger, ground, one tablespoon
- Coconut oil, two tablespoons
- Green cabbage, two cups shredded
- Butter, two tablespoons
- Yellow onion, minced, one half cup

BASIL SAUCE

- Mayonnaise, three-fourths cup
- Salt, one half teaspoon
- Black pepper, one half teaspoon
- Basil, fine chop, one tablespoon
- Radishes, one half cup sliced paper-thin

PICKLED ONION SALAD

- Rice vinegar, one tablespoon
- Scallions, one ounce
- Red chili pepper, one
- Salt, one half teaspoon
- Water, two tablespoons

Instructions

MEATBALLS: Heat oven to 200. Mix well all of the ingredients for the meatballs using a large spoon or your hands. Shape this mix into twenty little meatballs. Fry the meatballs in hot coconut oil for ten minutes. Put the meatballs in the oven to keep them warm. Fry the green cabbage in the melted butter over medium heat in a large skillet for ten minutes, stirring it occasionally. Arrange the cabbage on a plate and lay the meatballs on top of the cabbage. Serve the onion salad and the basil sauce on the side.

PICKLED ONION SALAD: Slice the chili pepper and the scallions thinly and mix them with the rice vinegar, water, and salt and set this mix to the side.

BASIL SAUCE: Mix the sliced radishes with the basil and the mayonnaise. Add in the salt and the pepper, mix well and set this to the side.

Nutrition per serving:

Calories 860, 9 grams net carbs, 77 grams fat, 30 grams protein

26. BACON BURGER CASSEROLE

Serves four

Ingredients:

- Ground beef, one pound
- Bacon, eight slices
- Tomatoes, two
- Dill pickles, two chopped fine
- Butter, one tablespoon
- Black pepper, one teaspoon
- Salt, one teaspoon
- Cheddar cheese, shredded, one cup
- Heavy cream, one cup
- Tomato paste, two tablespoons
- Eggs, two
- Garlic, minced, one tablespoon

Instructions

Heat the oven to 400. Fry the bacon in one tablespoon of butter for five minutes and chop into small pieces. Dump the chopped bacon back in the skillet and add in the ground beef and fry for an additional ten minutes until the beef is browned. Stir in two-thirds of the shredded cheese along with the tomatoes, the minced garlic, the seasonings, and the diced dill pickle. Use two tablespoons of lard to grease an eight by eight-inch baking pan. Mix the tomato paste, eggs, and cream in a small bowl and stir this into the meat mixture in the skillet. Put all of this mix into the baking pan and top it with the remainder of the shredded cheese. Bake for twenty minutes.

Nutrition per serving:

Calories 1041, 8 grams net carbs, 91 grams fat, 46 grams protein

27. SALMON WITH SPINACH AND PESTO

Serves four

Ingredients:

- Salmon, two pounds
- Parmesan cheese, grated, two ounces
- Pesto, green or red, one tablespoon
- Butter, one tablespoon
- Spinach, fresh, one pound
- Black pepper, one teaspoon
- Salt, one half teaspoon
- Sour cream, one cup

Instructions

Heat the oven to 400. Use two tablespoons of lard to grease a nine by a thirteen-inch baking pan. Season the salmon pieces with the salt and pepper and lay it in the baking pan with the skin down. Blend the sour cream, pesto, and parmesan cheese in a small bowl and use this mixture to coat the salmon. Bake the fish for twenty minutes. While the salmon is baking fry the spinach in the butter until it wilts, about two to three minutes. Serve the spinach with the baked salmon.

Nutrition per serving:

Calories 902, 3 grams net carbs, 78 grams fat, 45 grams protein

28. PEPPERONI PIZZA

Serves four

Ingredients:

- Pepperoni, sliced, four ounces
- Mozzarella, shredded, one and one half cups
- Tomato sauce, one cup
- Salt, one half teaspoon
- Cream of tartar, one quarter teaspoon
- Garlic powder, one teaspoon
- Whey protein powder, plain, one cup
- Eggs, three large beaten
- Water, one tablespoon
- Heavy cream, two tablespoons
- Butter, one quarter cup melted
- Cream cheese, eight ounces at room temperature

Instructions

Heat the oven to 350. Use two tablespoons of lard to grease a twelve-inch cast-iron skillet. Cream together the eggs, water, heavy cream, butter, and cream cheese. Add in the cream of tartar, salt, garlic powder, baking powder, and the protein powder. Blend all of this until it is smooth and then put it in the skillet and spread it to cover the bottom. Bake this for twenty minutes. Cover the crust with the tomato sauce, then top with the shredded cheese and add the pepperoni. Put the skillet of pizza back in the oven and bake for another ten minutes. Let the pizza cool for five minutes before cutting it.

Nutrition per serving:

Calories 300, 2.5 grams net carbs, 27.5 grams fat, 18.5 grams protein

29. AVOCADO SHRIMP SALAD

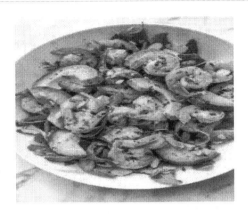

Serves four

Ingredients:

- Shrimp, one pound small size cooked, peeled, and deveined
- Cilantro, chopped fresh, two tablespoons
- Red onion, diced, one quarter cup
- Tomato, one small diced small
- Avocado, one peeled, pitted and diced
- Salt, one teaspoon
- Black pepper, one teaspoon
- Olive oil, one teaspoon
- Lime juice, one quarter cup

Instructions

Mix well the olive oil, lime juice, salt, and pepper in a medium-size bowl. Mix in the cilantro, red onion, tomato, avocado, and shrimp and mix it together well. This salad needs to be kept chilled until you are ready to serve it.

Nutrition per serving:

Calories 255, 4 grams net carbs, 13 grams fat, 27 grams protein

30. PHILLY CHEESE STEAK

Serves four

Ingredients:

- Sirloin steak, one pound
- Provolone cheese, four slices
- Sweet onion, one small sliced paper-thin
- Green pepper, one medium cleaned and sliced thin
- Salt, one teaspoon
- Black pepper, one teaspoon
- Olive oil, one tablespoon
- Keto bread, four slices

Instructions

Salt and pepper the steak and slice it into very thin strips, about one-eighth of an inch thick. Fry the steak strips in the olive oil over medium heat and cook until they are browned, five to ten minutes. Take the steak from the skillet and add in the green peppers and the onion and fry for five minutes. Lay a slice of cheese on a slice of keto bread and top with the steak slices and the onion and green pepper mixture.

Nutrition per serving:

Calories 350, 2.5 grams net carbs, 18 grams fat, 42 grams protein

Chapter Nine

SNACKS AND APPETIZERS

While the keto lifestyle does not encourage snacking between meals, there are times when you want a little something to hold you until the next meal. Or you might not be hungry enough for a full meal and a little snack will do just fine. And everyone would love to impress their guests or coworkers with a fabulous tray of goodies that they can also enjoy guilt-free. These snacks and appetizers will fit any of those situations.

1. BACON-WRAPPED SCALLOPS

Serves four

Ingredients:

- Salt, one half teaspoon
- Black pepper, one half teaspoon
- Olive oil, two tablespoons
- Bacon, eight slices cut in half, middle of the slice
- Sea scallops, sixteen
- Toothpicks, sixteen

Instructions

Heat the oven to 425. Lay parchment paper on a cookie sheet. Remove any side muscles the scallops might have and dry them with a paper towel. Use one half of a slice of bacon to wrap each scallop around and then hold the bacon to the scallop with a toothpick. Brush on the olive oil and then season with the salt and pepper. Lay the scallops on the parchment paper and bake for fifteen minutes.

Nutrition per serving:

Calories 224, 2 grams net carbs, 17 grams fat, 12 grams protein

2. BUFFALO CHICKEN JALAPENO POPPERS

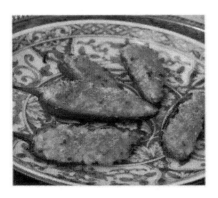

Serves five

Ingredients:

- Bacon, four slices cooked, drained, and crumbled
- Buffalo wing sauce, one quarter cup
- Mozzarella cheese, shredded, one quarter cup
- Blue cheese, crumbled, one half cup divided
- Cream cheese, four ounces at room temperature
- Salt, one half teaspoon
- Onion powder, one half teaspoon
- Garlic, minced, two tablespoons
- Chicken, ground, eight ounces
- Jalapeno peppers, ten large sizes, cut in half longways and seeds removed
- Ranch dressing and sliced green onions for serving

Instructions

Heat the oven to 350. Lay foil or parchment paper on a cookie sheet. Lay the jalapeno pepper halves on the foil or parchment paper. Cook together over medium heat the garlic, ground chicken, onion powder, and salt for about ten minutes until the chicken is fully cooked. Dump this mixture into a large bowl and mix in the wing sauce, mozzarella cheese, and one-quarter cup of the crumbled blue cheese. Put some of this mix into all of the pepper halves and top them with the bacon crumbles and the rest of the blue cheese. Bake the poppers for thirty minutes and serve with the ranch dressing and the green onions.

Nutrition for four poppers:

Calories 252, 4.6 grams net carbs, 19 grams fat, 16 grams protein

3. RUTABAGA FRIES

Serves eight

Ingredients:

- Rutabagas, two medium-sized about twenty-four ounces each
- Black pepper, one half teaspoon
- Salt, one teaspoon
- Olive oil, one quarter cup

Instructions

Heat the oven to 400. Wash and peel the rutabagas and slice them into one-quarter-inch thick circles. Slice each circle into sticks that are a one-quarter inch wide. Mix in a large bowl the sticks of rutabaga with the black pepper, salt, and olive oil. Arrange the fries on a metal rack that is sitting on top of a cookie sheet and back them for forty-five minutes.

Nutrition info per ten fries:

Calories 96, 6 grams net carbs, 6 grams fat, 1-gram protein

4. SPICY DEVILED EGGS

Makes twenty-four egg halves

Ingredients:

- Chives, minced, one teaspoon
- Chili powder, one teaspoon
- Salt, one teaspoon
- Black pepper, one teaspoon
- Dijon mustard, one tablespoon
- Sriracha sauce, one tablespoon
- Mayonnaise, one third cup
- Eggs, twelve larges

Instructions

Hard boil the eggs and when they are cool, peel them and cut them in half the long way. Remove the yolks gently and place them into a large bowl. Mash the yolks into a paste with a fork or a potato masher. Stir in the mustard, sriracha sauce, salt, pepper, chili powder, and the mayonnaise until the mix is smooth and creamy. Refill the egg whites with this mixture using a spoon or a frosting bag to pipe the mix in. When you are ready to serve the eggs top them with the chives.

Nutrition per egg half:

Calories 53, 1-gram net carbs, 4 grams fat, 2 grams protein

5. PESTO BACON AND CAPRESE SALAD SKEWERS

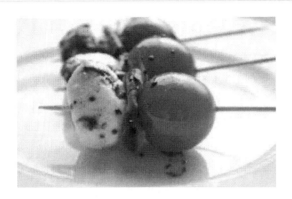

Serves 10, three skewers each

Ingredients:

- Black pepper, one teaspoon
- Salt, one teaspoon
- Olive oil, two tablespoons
- Basil pesto, one quarter cup
- Mozzarella balls or chunks, thirty pieces equaling ten ounces
- Basil, fresh, thirty leaves
- Bacon, five slices cooked and cut into six pieces each
- Grape tomatoes, thirty
- Toothpicks

Instructions

Place the food on the toothpicks in this order: mozzarella balls, basil leaf, bacon piece, and grape tomato. Mix together in a small bowl the olive oil and the pesto and drizzle it over the skewers and then sprinkle them with salt and pepper.

Nutrition info per three skewers:

Calories 153, 2 grams net carbs, 12 grams fat, 7 grams protein

6. BAKED COCONUT SHRIMP

Serves four

Ingredients:

- Black pepper, one half teaspoon
- Salt, one half teaspoon
- Paprika, one quarter teaspoon
- Garlic powder, one quarter teaspoon
- Coconut flakes, unsweetened, two cups
- Eggs, three large well beat
- Coconut flour, three tablespoons
- Medium shrimp, one pound, forty-two to forty-eight peeled and deveined, thawed

Instruction

Heat the oven to 400. Lay a wire rack onto a cookie sheet and spray it with oil spray. Set three bowls on the counter. In the first one put the beaten eggs, in the next one put the coconut flakes, and in the last one put a mix of the pepper, salt, paprika, garlic powder, and coconut flour. Dip each shrimp into the flour mixture first, then into the egg wash and then roll in the flakes of coconut. Lay them on the wire rack and bake for ten minutes, turning them over after five minutes.

Nutrition info:

Calories 443, 5 grams net carbs, 30 grams fat, 31 grams protein

7. BAKED GARLIC PARMESAN WINGS

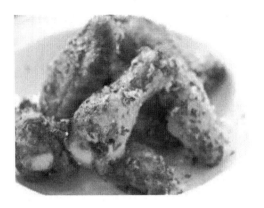

Serves six

Ingredients:

- Black pepper, one half teaspoons
- Salt, one teaspoon
- Onion powder, one teaspoon
- Garlic powder, two teaspoon
- Parsley, chopped, one tablespoon
- Garlic, minced, one tablespoon
- Parmesan cheese, grated, one half cup
- Butter, melted, one half cup
- Baking powder, two tablespoons
- Chicken wings, two pounds thawed

Instructions

Heat the oven to 250. Salt and pepper the wings and let them sit for ten minutes. Shake the baking powder over the wings and toss them so that the baking powder covers all of the wings. Spread the

191

wings on an oven rack and bake them for thirty minutes. Change the temperature of the oven to 425 and bake the wings for another thirty minutes. Prepare the sauce for the wings while the wings are baking by mixing the onion powder, garlic powder, parsley, minced garlic, parmesan cheese, and melted butter in a bowl. When the wings have finished cooking, let them sit for five minutes and then toss them in the sauce.

Nutrition info:

Calories 468, 2 grams carbs, 38 grams fat, 30 grams protein

8. COLD CRAB DIP

Serves twelve

Ingredients:

- Chives, chopped, two tablespoons
- Crabmeat, eight ounces, press between paper towels to remove any moisture
- Old Bay seasoning, one quarter to one half teaspoon (to taste)
- Lemon juice, one teaspoon
- Sour cream, three tablespoons
- Cream cheese, four ounces at room temperature

Instructions

Cream together the lemon juice, seasoning, sour cream, and cream cheese until smooth and creamy. Gently fold in the chives and the crab meat just until mixed with the cream cheese mixture. Serve with slices of bell pepper, cucumber, or celery.

Nutrition info:

Calories 41, 0 grams net carbs, 2 grams fat, 3 grams protein

9. CHICKEN NUGGETS

Serves four

Ingredients:

- Butter, four tablespoons
- Black pepper, one half teaspoon
- Salt, one teaspoon
- Garlic powder, one teaspoon
- Onion powder, one teaspoon
- Paprika, one teaspoon
- Tapioca flour, one tablespoon
- Coconut flour, three tablespoons
- Chicken breast or tenders, one pound skinless and boneless cut into chunks

Instructions

Heat the oven to 425. Mix together in a large bowl the tapioca flour, coconut flour, salt, pepper, onion garlic, and paprika. Melt the butter and put it into a shallow pan. Coat the chicken pieces with the melted butter and then roll them in the flour mixture. Bake the nuggets for fifteen minutes, turning after eight minutes.

Nutrition info:

Calories 252, 4.2 grams net carbs, 13 grams fat, 27 grams protein

10. ONION RINGS

Serves two

Ingredients:

- Parmesan cheese, grated, one half cup
- Pork rinds, crushed, one half cup
- Heavy whipping cream, one tablespoon
- Eggs, two large
- Coconut flour, one half cup
- Onion, one white medium-sized

Instructions

Heat the oven to 425. Slice the onion into one half-inch thick rings after peeling it. You will need three different bowls for the dipping of the onion rings. Place the coconut flour in the first bowl, the mixed whipping cream and beaten egg in the second bowl, and the mixed pork rinds and parmesan cheese in the last bowl. Dip the onion rings in the flour, then the egg wash, and then the pork rind mix. Bake the onion ring in the oven for fifteen minutes.

Nutrition info:

Calories 211, 4.5 grams net carbs, 12.5 grams fat, 16 grams protein

11. SAUSAGE STUFFED MUSHROOMS

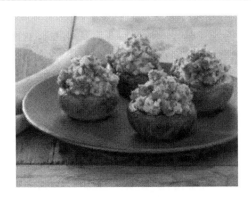

Makes twenty mushrooms

Ingredients:

- Sausage, two links any type
- Baby Bella Mushrooms, twenty
- Cheddar Cheese, one cup
- Onion, diced, one quarter cup
- Garlic, minced, two teaspoons
- Black pepper, one half teaspoon
- Salt, one half teaspoon
- Butter, two tablespoons

Instructions

Heat the oven to 350. Wash and dry the mushrooms. Pull the stalks off and chop the stalks up finely. Mix the diced stalks with the diced onions. Pull off the casing from the sausage and throw it away. Cook the sausage meat in the two tablespoons of butter in a skillet over medium heat. When the sausage is fully cooked, take it from the pan and set it aside. Put the garlic, mushroom stalks, and diced onion into the pan with the leftover liquid and cook for five minutes, stirring often. Pour this mix into a bowl and add the salt, pepper, cheddar cheese, and sausage. Fill all of the mushroom caps with the sausage mixture. Set the caps on a cookie sheet and bake the mushrooms for twenty minutes.

Nutrition info per mushroom:

Calories 56, 1.3 grams net carbs, 3.7 grams fat, 3.3 grams protein

12. PARMESAN CRISPS

Serves two

Ingredients:

- Jalapeno, one medium (optional)
- Provolone cheese, two slices
- Parmesan cheese, grated, eight tablespoons

Instructions

Heat the oven to 425. Lay parchment paper on a cookie sheet. Lay eight mounds of parmesan, one tablespoon each, on the parchment paper. If you are using the jalapeno clean out the seeds and slice the pepper as thin or as thick as you want to. Lay these slices on the parmesan cheese. Cut the slices of mozzarella into four equal squares and lay one square over the parmesan cheese and the jalapeno if you are using it. Bake these for nine minutes and allow to cool slightly before eating. These are great served with ranch dressing or sour cream.

Nutrition info per crisp:

Calories 162, 1.5 grams carbs, 10 grams fat, 14 grams protein

13. ZUCCHINI PIZZA BITES

Serves six

Ingredients:

- Pepperoni, one quarter cup mini slices

- Mozzarella cheese, one cup

- Provolone cheese, grated, one half cup

- Black pepper, one quarter teaspoon

- Salt, one half teaspoon

- Italian seasoning, one teaspoon

- Egg, one

- Zucchini, shredded, two cups

Instructions

Heat the oven to 400. Use olive oil cooking spray to spray a mini muffin pan. Lay the shredded zucchini in paper towels and squeeze out as much liquid as possible. Dump the shredded zucchini into a bowl and add the provolone cheese, salt, pepper, Italian seasoning, and egg, mixing thoroughly. Divide the mixture into the muffin cups, packing the mix down into each cup. Sprinkle the mozzarella cheese onto the cups and then top the cheese with the mini pepperonis. Bake them for fifteen to eighteen minutes. Let them sit for ten minutes before serving, using a butter knife to loosen them from the pan.

Nutrition per serving:

Calories 230, 3 grams net carbs, 9.3 grams fat, 16.4 grams fat

14. TUNA IN CUCUMBER CUPS

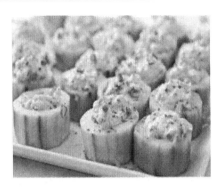

Makes ten

Ingredients:

- Dill, fresh for garnish
- Black pepper, one teaspoon
- Mayonnaise, one third cup
- Tuna, one six-ounce can
- Cucumber, one large cut into one-inch thick slices

Instructions

Use a small spoon or a melon baller to scoop most of the middle out of the slices of cucumber, leaving just a thin line at the bottom to make the cup. Put the cucumber you removed into a paper towel and press it to remove excess liquid. Chop the cucumber finely and put it into a bowl with the drained tuna, mayonnaise, and pepper. Mix this well and use a small spoon to fill the cucumber cups. Garnish with a sprig of fresh dill and serve.

Nutrition info per cup:

Calories 22, 2 grams net carbs, .7 grams fat, 2 grams protein

15. ITALIAN SUB ROLL-UPS

Serves four

Ingredients:

- Italian seasoning
- Apple cider vinegar
- Olive oil
- Lettuce, shredded
- Mayonnaise
- Provolone cheese, four slices
- Pepperoni, four slices
- Sopressata, four slices
- Mortadella, four slices
- Genoa salami, four slices
- Toothpicks

Instructions

Layout the largest slices of meat first. Then add the next smallest slices, going until all of the meat is in four stacks. Spread mayonnaise thinly on the meat, staying near the center, so it does not ooze out when you roll it up. Lay the slices of provolone cheese on the stacks. Add in some of the shredded lettuce and season with the Italian seasoning. Roll up the stacks and hold with a toothpick. Drizzle the rolls with the apple cider vinegar and the olive oil.

Nutrition info per roll:

Calories 235, 1 gram net carbs, 20 grams fat, 10 grams protein

Chapter Ten

SAUCES AND DRESSINGS

Many sauces and dressings can be store-bought but they might also have added sugars, and they will certainly have added preservatives that you may be trying to eliminate from your diet. Any sauce or dressing can be easily made at home with fresh ingredients.

1. LOW CARB STRAWBERRY JAM

Ingredients:

- Knox gelatin powder, three-fourths teaspoon
- Lemon juice, one tablespoon
- Water, one quarter cup
- Sugar replacement, one quarter cup
- Strawberries, diced, one cup

Instructions

Sprinkle the lemon juice with the gelatin and allow it to sit and thicken. Add the water, strawberries, and sugar replacement to a small pot and set it over medium heat. As soon as this mixture begins to simmer then lower the heat and let it simmer for twenty minutes. Chop up the gelatin lemon juice mix and mix it in with the warm strawberries and let it dissolve. Let the jam cool after removing the pan from the heat, then spoon the mix into a clean glass jar. This jam will remain good in the refrigerator for two weeks.

This can be made with any low carb fruit.

Nutrition info per tablespoon:

Calories 57, .85 grams net carbs, 0 grams fat, .66 grams protein

2. PLAIN MAYONNAISE

Ingredients:

- Lemon juice, two teaspoons
- Olive oil, one cup
- Dijon mustard, one tablespoon at room temperature
- Egg yolk, one at room temperature

Instructions

Cream together the mustard and the egg yolk and then pour in the oil slowly while stirring to mix. Add in the lemon juice and mix one last time and then let the mixture sit until it is thick. This will keep for about four days in the refrigerator.

Nutrition info per one quarter cup:

Calories 511, 0 grams net carbs, 57 grams fat, 1 gram protein

3. RANCH DIP

Ingredients:

- Ranch seasoning, two tablespoons
- Sour cream, one half cup
- Mayonnaise, one cup

Instructions

Mix all of the ingredients together and allow to chill for at least one hour before serving.

Nutrition info one quarter cup:

Calories 241, 1-gram net carbs, 26 grams fat, 1 gram protein

4. AVOCADO SAUCE

Ingredients:

- Pistachio nuts, two ounces
- Salt, one teaspoon
- Lime juice, one quarter cup
- Garlic, minced, two tablespoons
- Water, one quarter cup
- Olive oil, two-thirds cup
- Avocado, one
- Parsley or cilantro, fresh, one cup

Instructions

Use a food processor or a blender to mix all of the ingredients together until they are smooth except the pistachio nuts and olive oil. Ad these at the end and mix well. If the mix is a bit thick add in a bit more oil or water. This sauce will stay fresh in the refrigerator for up to four days.

Nutrition info per quarter cup:

Calories 490, 5 grams net carbs, 50 grams fat, 5 grams protein

5. BLUE CHEESE DRESSING

Ingredients:

- Parsley, fresh, two tablespoons
- Black pepper, one teaspoon
- Salt, one teaspoon
- Heavy whipping cream, one half cup
- Mayonnaise, one half cup
- Greek yogurt, three-fourths cup
- Blue cheese, five ounces

Instructions

Break the blue cheese up into small chunks in a large bowl. Stir in the heavy cream, mayonnaise, and yogurt. Mix in the parsley, salt, and pepper and let the dressing sit for one hour, so the flavors mix well. This dressing will be good in the refrigerator for three days.

Nutrition per one quarter cup:

Calories 477, 4 grams net carbs, 47 grams fat, 10 grams protein

6. SALSA DRESSING

Ingredients:

- Garlic, minced, one tablespoon
- Chili powder, one teaspoon
- Apple cider vinegar, three tablespoons
- Mayonnaise, two tablespoons
- Sour cream, two tablespoons
- Olive oil, one quarter cup
- Salsa, one half cup

Instructions

Add all of the ingredients to a large bowl and mix well. Pour into a glass jar and let the dressing chill in the refrigerator for at least one hour. This dressing will stay good in the refrigerator for three days.

Nutrition per one quarter cup:

Calories 200, 2 grams net carbs, 21 grams fat, 1-gram protein

7. GUACAMOLE

Ingredients:

- Salt, one half teaspoon
- Black pepper, one teaspoon
- Garlic, minced, one tablespoon
- Cilantro, four tablespoons
- Olive oil, two tablespoons
- Tomato, one diced small
- Lime juice, two tablespoons
- White onion, one half chopped finely
- Avocado, two ripe

Instructions

Wash, peel, and pit the avocados and mash the pulp with a fork. Stir in the garlic, salt, pepper, cilantro, olive oil, tomato, lime juice, and onion. Let the guacamole sit for at least two hours before serving.

Nutrition info one quarter cup:

Calories 238, 5 grams net carbs, 22 grams fat, 3 grams protein

8. SPICY PIMIENTO CHEESE

Ingredients:

- Cheddar cheese, shredded, one half cup
- Cayenne pepper, one eighth teaspoon
- Dijon mustard, one tablespoon
- Paprika, one teaspoon
- Chili powder, one teaspoon
- Pimientos, finely chopped, four tablespoons
- Mayonnaise, one third cup

Instructions

Cream all of the ingredients together and then refrigerate for at least one hour before serving. This cheese will stay good in the refrigerator for up to five days.

Nutrition info one quarter cup:

Calories 248, 1 gram net carbs, 24 grams fat, 7 grams protein

9. CAESAR DRESSING

Ingredients:

- Lemon juice, one tablespoon
- Anchovies, one ounce
- Salt, one half teaspoon
- Garlic, minced, one teaspoon
- Black pepper, one quarter teaspoon
- Apple cider vinegar, one teaspoon
- Dijon mustard, one tablespoon
- Olive oil, one half cup
- Parmesan cheese, grated, one quarter cup

Instructions

Blend together all of the ingredients. If the dressing seems to be a little too thick then add drops of water until it is the right consistency. This dressing will stay good in the refrigerator for up to three days.

Nutrition info per one quarter cup:

Calories 298, 1 gram net carbs, 31 grams fat, 6 grams protein

10. HUMMUS

Ingredients:

- Black pepper, one half teaspoon
- Salt, one half teaspoon
- Cumin, ground, one half teaspoon
- Garlic, minced, one tablespoon
- Lemon juice, two tablespoons
- Tahini, one quarter cup
- Sunflower seeds, one quarter cup
- Olive oil, one half cup
- Cilantro, fresh chopped, one half cup
- Avocados, three ripe

Instructions

Wash, dry, and peel the avocados. Take out the pits and drop the flesh into a food processor or a blender with the remainder of the ingredients. Mix everything well until the mix is smooth and creamy.

Nutrition info per quarter cup:

Calories 417, 4 grams net carbs, 41 grams fat, 5 grams protein

Chapter Eleven

SEVEN DAY MEAL PLAN

This is a sample seven-day meal plan for you to follow. This is only a suggestion and you should feel free to substitute any of the menu ideas for other menu items. All of these recipes are found in this book.

DAY ONE	
Breakfast	Cauliflower Hash Browns
Lunch	Pepperoni Pizza
Dinner	Tuna Casserole
DAY TWO	
Breakfast	Smoked Salmon Sandwich
Lunch	Tex Mex Stuffed Zucchini Boats
Dinner	Avocado Shrimp Boats
DAY THREE	
Breakfast	Coconut Porridge
Lunch	Deviled Egg Salad
Dinner	Bacon Wrapped Meatloaf
DAY FOUR	
Breakfast	Oatmeal
Lunch	Sloppy Joes
Dinner	White Fish with Curry and Coconut
DAY FIVE	
Breakfast	Scrambled Eggs with Halloumi Cheese

Lunch	Baked Fish Sticks
Dinner	Herbed Grilled Chicken
DAY SIX	
Breakfast	Mushroom Omelet
Lunch	Chicken Cabbage and Onions
Dinner	Spinach and Goat Cheese Pie
DAY SEVEN	
Breakfast	Coconut Cream with Berries
Lunch	Pigs in a Blanket
Dinner	Chicken Bacon Ranch Casserole

Chapter Twelve

SPICES FOR KETO COOKING

Your keto cooking will never be boring if you learn to use spices to flavor your food. Here is a list of common spices that you can experiment with to add in some flavor to the dishes you create.

Allspice: This single spice gives the flavor of cinnamon, nutmeg and cloves. It is usually used ground in recipes for poultry, seafood and meat marinades.

Basil: The sweet yet peppery taste of basil in used in pesto and almost always in any dish that contains tomatoes. Basil also works well with rosemary, parsley, thyme, oregano, and sage.

Bay Leaves: Potently flavored, just a leaf or two of bay will usually suffice in marinades for meats and poultry. It's even found in an occasional dessert.

Chives: These are a part of the onion family but they are milder and more delicate in flavor. They work well in salads and egg dishes.

Cilantro: A strongly aromatic seasoning that has a pungent flavor reminiscent of sage and lemon.

Cinnamon: This adds a warm spiciness to food. It complements meats and vegetables like carrots, spinach, and onions. Cinnamon is often used with other warm spices, like allspice, ginger, cardamom, nutmeg, cloves and pepper.

Cloves: Cloves are often used as a flavoring for meat dishes. This spice also works well with black pepper, ginger, nutmeg, and cinnamon.

Coriander: This spice is often used to flavor meat, poultry, and vegetable dishes. It has an orangey scent and tastes sweet and warm.

Cumin: This spice works well in recipes for eggs, seafood, meats and poultry, as well as sauces that are tomato based.

Garlic: This is a versatile seasoning that complements most any savory dish. Garlic can be used to flavor almost any dish.

Ginger: This spice works well in sauces and stir fries, especially any dish with an Asian flair.

Marjoram: This is a relative of oregano with but with a lighter, more delicate flavor. It works well with many vegetables, poultry and meats.

Nutmeg: This spice is used in recipes for seafood, poultry, eggs, cheeses, and vegetables (especially eggplant, spinach, and cabbage).

Onion: These come in many varieties and sizes and can be used anywhere you want to use them.

Oregano: Oregano is related to marjoram, but its flavor is stronger. You will usually find it in tomato-based recipes. It pairs up well with other spices, like thyme, garlic, basil, and parsley.

Paprika: This spice is used in vegetable dishes as well as eggs and poultry. It is especially useful as a garnish due to its beautiful color.

Parsley: Parsley is used in meat marinades, dressings, salads, casseroles, and omelets.

Pepper: This spice comes in ground black pepper and the lighter flavored ground white pepper.

Rosemary: This spice is used liberally in marinades and with roasted and grilled foods, like vegetables, poultry, and seafood.

Sage: Sage has a pungent, slightly bitter/sweet taste and an herbal fragrance. It is especially good in meats, seafood, poultry, and dressings.

Thyme: This is a pungent seasoning that has a minty flavor and scent. Try it, lightly in the beginning, with meat, seafood, poultry, and in marinades.

Conclusion

Thank you for making it through to the end of *Keto for Women Over 50*, let's hope it was informative and able to provide you with all of the tools you need to achieve your goals whatever they may be.

The next step is to make the commitment to follow the keto lifestyle and begin your journey to a new and better life. While you might be a woman over 50 you still have a lot of life to live and you should be able to live that life to the fullest. And that will begin with the best possible nutrition that will give you the health and the ability to be active that will carry you into the next phase of your life.

Finally, if you found this book useful in any way, a review on Amazon is always appreciated!

Intermittent Fasting for Women Over 50

(and not only)

JULIA CHRISTEN

Introduction

Whether you are hoping to lose weight or gain health benefits, many fad diets that claim they can help. Yet, these fads are nothing more than crash diets that cause a person to lose weight overly quickly in an unsustainable manner. The result? A woman may temporarily lose weight, but, before long, they gain even more weight back as the crash diet damaged their metabolism. Many women fifty and over have had their fair share of these diets, whether it is Weight Watchers, the South Beach Diet, Atkins, or worse yet, even more, extreme options such as the lemonade diet. After years of attempting to gain health and lose weight, many women are left worse off than they started.

Fear not; there is a solution. There is a way to lose weight that is not a crash diet. With intermittent fasting, which has been practiced for centuries all across the world, you can boost your health and rev up your metabolism for the ultimate form of maintainable and lasting weight loss.

Intermittent fasting allows your body to go through the eating cycles it is designed for. The human body has gone through these eating cycles naturally during periods of the day and night throughout history. Whether for religious reasons or only as a basic pattern to everyday life, these short terms of fasting allow the body to burn off the calories you have stored and use the break-in eating to heal itself. Intermittent fasting is great for adults of all ages, but especially for women as they age as it can help their metabolism to recover from years of dieting culture, as well as treating common age-related ailments such as high blood pressure, insulin resistance, and more.

By starting your journey with intermittent fasting, you can enjoy all your favorite foods, experience more energy, increased health, and maintainable weight loss. Within the pages of this book, you will find everything you need to get started and then some.

Chapter One

WHAT IS INTERMITTENT FASTING?

Intermittent fasting, otherwise known as short-term fasting, is different than the long hours of fasting that comes to many peoples' minds when they hear the word "fasting." While long hours of fasting frequently cause intense hunger, weakness, and deprive the body of essential nutrients, the same is not true of intermittent fasting. With this form of fasting, your body still gains all the nutrients and calories it requires, but it also harnesses the body's natural metabolism to its fullest to increase health and weight loss.

It may seem foreign to practice intermittent fasting, but the truth is that humans already practice short-term fasting while sleeping. That is where the word "breakfast" originates, as it is the meal that breaks our overnight fast. The human body is formed in such a way that periods of short-term fasting allow our health and metabolism to reach its peak. Yet, many people in today's modern society snack and graze, never utilizing the benefits that intermittent fasting has to offer.

Fasting has a long history in everyday practice, medicine, and even religion throughout the world. In this chapter, we will examine intermittent fasting and its roots throughout history so that you can fully understand how to harness it and gain all the benefits it has to offer, both to your health and to your waistline.

While previous health theories before the age of science were not always accurate or helpful, science has recently found that many of these practices have a solid basis. The doctors prescribing various practices for healing may not have understood the science behind why something worked, such as in ancient Chinese medicine, but science is slowly examining these practices and coming to know why they are so useful. One shining example of this is intermittent fasting. Many ancient cultures and religions would prescribe fasting for people who were of poor health, and now through scientific studies, researchers have found that intermittent fasting does have healing proprieties. One of the most famous physicians that prescribed fasting during ancient history was Hippocrates from Greece.

Fasting has also been practiced for religious purposes for centuries. Not only have humans used fasting for religion and health, but it was also a necessary aspect of daily life throughout history. Before modern times, many people would be out working in the fields, workshops, or anywhere else they could make a living. Due to this, they were unable to stop and eat quickly. Instead, the time between their meals would lengthen, turning into a valid fasting window. This intermittent fasting, while not intentional, allowed individuals to attain the health and weight benefits that fasting has to offer. Sadly, due to modern amenities, many people no longer practice regular short-term fasting. But, with the new scientific understanding of intermittent fasting's benefits, more people are beginning to go back to this healthy and natural way of life.

As you can see from the religious fasting examples, there are many different types of fasting. Some individuals abstain from all food and drink, others only abstain from food, and sometimes only specific foods are off-limits. Intermittent fasting is a moderate example of fasting in which a person refrains from all food but is free to enjoy any calorie-free drinks. Although, there are a few forms of intermittent fasting that do allow a person to consume a limited number of calories over a more extended period. We will discuss this fasting in-depth later on.

Intermittent fasting is an effective weight loss option as it not only limits your caloric intake, but it also boosts your metabolism, so you burn off more calories and body fat. Most of the time, humans eat so frequently that our bodies are continually attempting to burn off the calories we have recently eaten. But, when you practice intermittent fasting, you give your body that opportunity to burn off body fat instead of a snack, thereby allowing you to lose weight.

Even if you eat a low-calorie snack, you will likely be adding to your body weight. This is because your body can only hold a certain amount of glucose at one time, and once your glucose reserves in your muscles and liver are full, the body must transform the remaining glucose into lipids, which are stored as body fat. Since low-calorie snacks are made with carbohydrates, which is glucose, whenever you graze on these snacks during the day, you impede your weight loss.

On the other hand, if you eat a large calorie-dense and nutritious meal that will keep you satisfied, you can go all day without eating. This will not only lower your daily calorie intake, but it will also allow you to burn off the calories you consumed in your meal plus your body fat, reducing your weight at a manageable and healthy rate.

There are multiple types of intermittent fasting, which allows a person to find the exact version that is right for their lifestyle. Unlike diets that make you change your lifestyle to lose weight, you will find that intermittent fasting can seamlessly fit into most lifestyles. You can customize the approach to best work for you. There is no need to miss out on dining out with family, going out drinking with friends, or enjoying your favorite foods in moderation.

For instance, if you typically enjoy going out to eat with family and friends in the evening, you can begin your fasting after your last meal or drink, and then fast until noon the following day. This will allow you to enjoy your healthy lifestyle while still practicing intermittent fasting. As many people do not feel hungry in the morning, this is a common approach to intermittent fasting. Of course, you can choose any time of day to fast that best works for you, and you can customize your fasting window length.

When you take up intermittent fasting, you shouldn't have to obsess over food or when you eat or don't eat. You shouldn't be staring at the clock hungry and tired, waiting for your next meal. Instead, you can listen to your body, eat when you are hungry, and go without when you are satisfied. Of course, when you first begin intermittent fasting, there will be an adjustment period, but you can make this easier on yourself by slowly altering your usual eating habits. For instance, if you usually eat every four or six hours, you can gradually increase the time between meals by thirty minutes. By increasing your fasting window by only thirty minutes at a time, you won't suffer from hunger pangs or fatigue, but you will allow your body to adjust to a fasting lifestyle slowly.

When you begin intermittent fasting, it is essential to remember that you don't only increase the time between your meals, but you also eat healthier meals that are calorie-dense. By eating a large number of healthy calories within a meal, you will be able to go more extended periods between eating while still staying satisfied and full.

While you can eat a regular healthy diet without any constrictions when practicing intermittent fasting, you can also increase the health and weight loss benefits by combining intermittent fasting with a ketogenic diet. The ketogenic diet is perfectly paired with intermittent fasting, as it prioritizes healthy and calorie-dense meals. Not only that, but as the ketogenic diet produces the fuel type known as "ketones," which are also produced when fasting, you will find that you experience increased energy.

You must understand that your body is not in a fasted state the entire time you are fasting. When you first finish a meal, your body is in a fed state, also known as the absorptive state, where it is working on breaking down the nutrients you have eaten. After a few hours, you enter the post-absorptive state, in which your body is working to use the food you have eaten as fuel. Lastly, after eight to twelve hours of not eating, you enter the fasted state. During the fasted state, you have burned off the calories from the food you have eaten, and your body will turn to use body fat as a fuel source, as well as producing ketones for fuel. While a short twelve-hour fast can give you health benefits, if you do not enter the fasted state until hour twelve of not eating, then you will only experience a small portion of the health and weight loss benefits intermittent fasting has to offer. On the other hand, a longer fasting window, such as a sixteen-hour fast, will give your body a long time to remain in a fasted state, allowing you to reap all the benefits intermittent fasting has to offer.

THE AUTOPHAGY PROCESS

Autophagy, pronounced as "aw-TOFF-uh-gee," is a vital human metabolic function. Sadly, this function can slow down as we age, causing health numerous health problems for women as they approach age fifty. But, what does autophagy mean? It is a combination of two Greek words, and when placed together, these words translate to "eat thyself."

Most laypeople still have very little to no understanding of the autophagy process, as researchers only began to understand the basics of it back in the 1950's. Yet, what these researchers learned is incredibly valuable. They found that there is a particular aspect of the cells within our bodies known as the organelle, specifically the lysosome organelle. Within the lysosome are enzymes whose express purpose is to aid in the digestion of fuel.

Later on, it was discovered that the lysosome organelle contains within them even smaller cells and organelles. But what does it mean? This shocking revelation spurred the researchers onward, and they found that there is a system, later named autophagosomes, that drive old and damaged cells to the lysosomes.

You may be wondering what the purpose of the autophagy system is and why the lysosome must consume other cells. When our cells become old and damaged, they are no longer able to function correctly. Therefore, the lysosome helps not only by consuming and getting rid of these cells but by recycling them to build and create younger and healthier cells that we can effectively use.

We all use the autophagy metabolic process in our daily lives in ways that we aren't even aware of. For instance, when we have been infected with a virus or bacteria after our immune system works on fighting back against the harmful properties, it is the autophagy process that helps to remove the toxic substances from our system.

This incredibly important system cannot be replicated by the use of prescription drugs, although researchers are seeking to find a way to activate it for the treatment of diseases. Yet, while you are not able to induce it with medication, there is another way to boost and increase your natural autophagy system: by practicing intermittent fasting. By triggering such an increase through fasting, women over fifty can begin to take back their health and prevent age-related diseases such as early-onset Alzheimer's diseases, type II diabetes, cancer, and more.

If you want to age well and feel young again, I can't stress enough the importance of the autophagy system and putting it to work for you.

Now that you have an understanding of the basics behind the fasting method, let's look at the main types of intermittent fasting.

THE 12/12 FAST

The perfect fasting method for beginners is the 12/12 fast, which is named such due to the twelve-hour feeding window and twelve-hour fasting window. When getting started, it may sound like going twelve hours without eating is a lot, but you likely already do this, at least some of the time. After all, if you finish eating your last meal of the day at 7 pm and then eat breakfast at 7 am, you have completed a twelve-hour fast!

If you are someone who habitually snacks late at night, try to prioritize eating more substantial nutrient and calorie-dense meals, which will keep you satisfied until your morning meal. Keep in mind that while this is a beautiful fast to get started with, you will want to try more advanced and longer fasting windows in the future. This is because the human body generally only enters the fasted state after twelve hours without eating, so you will only be able to gain a limited number of benefits with a short fast. To attain the full benefits of intermittent fasting, you will want to advance to a longer fast, such as the 16/8 fast, which will allow you to remain in the fasted state for several hours before eating.

THE 16/8 FAST

One of the most popular fasting methods is the 16/8 fast, named so due to the sixteen-hour fasting window and eight-hour eating window. This method is so popular, as it is simple to accomplish once you have adjusted to intermittent fasting with the 12/12 way. Due to its longer fasting window, you can experience all the benefits of intermittent fasting, as the human body enters the fasted state at around twelve hours after eating, meaning you can stay in the metabolic fasted state for approximately four hours before eating again.

You will find that this method is also known as the Leangains Method, and some people will customize it to have a shorter fasting window. Some women prefer to use a fourteen or fifteen-hour fast instead of the sixteen-hour, but it is all based on personal preference and ease.

While everyone can adjust this fast to their schedule, one common way to practice the 16/8 fast is simply by skipping breakfast. This is easy for many people who find that they are not hungry in the morning. But remember, to skip breakfast, you first have to ensure that you eat a large and healthy dinner the night before to help sustain you until lunchtime.

When lunchtime arrived, don't eat a small or unhealthy meal. Instead, you should focus on eating healthy and calorie-dense food that will refuel your energy and prepare you for the next time you fast.

THE 20/4 FAST

While a more extreme version of fasting, women who have adjusted to the 16/8 fasting method and want more of a challenge may desire to try the 20/4 fast. A large fluid intake must accompany the twenty hours of fasting during the fasting window. During your four-hour eating window, try to eat two large and calorie-dense meals, full of healthy nutrients. You will want these meals to contain your entire caloric, protein, and fat needs for the day.

This fast is often best started after lunchtime. By starting after lunch, you can enjoy a large breakfast, lunch, and maybe even a snack before you begin your fast. If you finish lunch at 12 pm, then your fast will go until the following day at 8 am, meaning you can eat your meals that day as usual.

If you find this fast is overly tricky when you first start, don't hesitate to cut it short. Instead of pushing yourself to finish the full twenty-hour fast, you can slowly increase your fasting window naturally until you get to your goal.

5:2 DAY FASTING

This method of fasting is the most intense that we describe here, as two days out of the week, a person fasts for nearly the entire day. You should not schedule your two fasting days together, but instead, have them separated by eating days. For instance, don't schedule your fast for both Tuesday and Wednesday. Alternatively, you should schedule them for Tuesday and Thursday so that you have a day in-between to eat plenty.

On fasting days, a person should generally consume only calorie-free drinks, such as water. But women are allowed five-hundred calories in food these days. This means you can have one large meal, prioritizing nutrients such as healthy proteins and fats. This method of fasting should be scheduled on days that are easiest for you. Most people choose to not fast on the weekends, as that is their time to enjoy themselves fully. Instead, weekdays, where you are at work or busy with errands, are often the best days to fast, as you will be too busy to think about eating.

While any of these fasting methods will work for women fifty and over, you want to prioritize a method ideal for the aging female body. While every woman is different, in general, the best option will be a fourteen to sixteen-hour fasting window. With this window, you can experience all benefits that a longer fasting window has to offer, but without the struggle of making it through a prolonged fasting window. You can enjoy slightly more frequent meals to keep your energy up, and still lose weight and boost your health.

Chapter Two

WHY INTERMITTENT FASTING IS IDEAL FOR WOMEN OVER 50

There are many benefits to intermittent fasting that make it ideal for women as they age. Not only do women struggle to lose weight as they get older, and their metabolism slows down, but they also are more prone to many age-related and weight-related diseases. In this chapter, we will go point-by-point on some of the best reasons to choose this lifestyle.

Weight Loss

While many people try diet after diet to lose weight, only to be disappointed, you can expect to find much more success with intermittent fasting. After all, while the human body is usually forced to be burning off the food regularly we have eaten, when you are in a fasted state, you can instead work on burning off your body fat. In the past, it was natural to go long periods without eating while working for the day. In today's modern society, we take a break for lunch and often for a snack as well, which only impedes weight loss. But, with fasting, you can eat the same number of calories and still lose weight, all because you are allowing your body to use the fat it has stored up.

Multiple studies conducted on intermittent fasting have found it much more effective than a variety of popular dieting and weight loss options, even when a person doesn't reduce their caloric intake.

Metabolic Reset

Many women, as they age, experience reduced metabolism. This is partly due to the natural aging process, and partly due to damaging the metabolism over the decades. Frequent crash dieting, poor sleep, overworking, poor health, and more can all damage your metabolism, thus preventing you from losing weight. But, by merely practicing intermittent fasting, you can reset and boost your metabolism, not only allowing you to lose weight but also helping you to feel healthier and maintain healthy lean muscle as you age.

Increase Human Growth Hormone

Hormones play an essential role in human health, something of which women are exceptionally aware of as they age. But many women are unaware of how to take advantage of the human growth hormone, also known as HGH. As this name implies, this hormone affects growth, but that is not all! This hormone is vital for bone health and density, cellular growth and regeneration, tissue health, and muscle mass. As women age, they tend to lose muscle mass, bones become thin and brittle, and cells begin to decay, increasing the speed of aging: all things that an increased level of HGH hormone can help improve.

When your body is in a fasted state, it leads to a boost in a natural increase in the HGH hormone. Studies have proven that this hormone can rise to five times its average level during a fast, meaning you can experience great full-body benefits to your health.

While it can be harmful if you experience a rise of this nature in many of your hormones, the same is not true of the human growth hormones. Studies have found that it is perfectly safe, even when it rises to this degree and higher. This is especially true since people naturally experience their HGH levels lowering as they age.

Convert Your Body Fat

Many people are unaware, but there are two types of body fat, white and brown. This fat is not created equal. Just as there is healthy and unhealthy cholesterol, there is also sturdy and unhealthy body fat. The white fat, which is what builds up as people gain excess weight, is damaging to health, contributes to aging, and leads to disease.

On the other hand, brown body fat is vital in protecting the body's inner organs and maintaining health. When you practice intermittent fasting, it not only helps you lose weight, but it can also actively convert your unhealthy white fat to healthy brown fat. As if that weren't good enough, brown fat also helps burn off white fat, meaning that the more brown fat you have, the more you will burn off excess white body fat.

Improve Muscle Health

Many people get excited about the temporary weight reduction they experience when trying the crash diet. That is until they stop losing weight and eventually give up on a diet. But, most of the weight loss people achieve on these diets is not fat loss but water weight and muscle weight. Muscle weighs more than fat, so even a small amount of muscle loss can make a big difference on the scale.

As crash diets promote malnutrition, it naturally leads to muscle loss, which negatively affects your health and strength as you age. After all, your muscles are in much more than your arms. They are surrounding your entire body, and even your heart is a muscle! As you lose muscle, your health and energy will be dramatically affected, and it is essential to regain this as you age if you want to improve your health. Thankfully, studies have found that when compared to dieting, intermittent fasting not only leads to more weight loss than dieting, but it also causes much less muscle loss. This means your muscles will become much healthier, especially if you actively workout while you practice fasting.

Boosted Energy

The mitochondria, which are within our mitochondrial cells, are the powerhouse of the cell. It is the mitochondria that allow us to use a variety of fuel sources from the food we eat as fuel, as well as ketones. While other cells in the body may only be able to utilize one or two fuel types for energy, the mitochondrial is incredibly versatile to be able to use all kinds of fuel. When you fast for longer periods (or are on a low-carb/ketogenic diet), your body begins to produce ketones, which are then used to cross the blood-brain barrier and fuel the brain in the absence of glucose. But that is not all. When you are in this fasted state of ketosis, the body will also increase the number of mitochondrial cells within your body, replacing non-mitochondrial cells with mitochondrial cells, allowing for more of your cells to be fueled by any fuel source.

Since the mitochondrial fuel ninety percent of the human body, by increasing the number of these cells, you can naturally increase your energy. Not only will your physical energy increase, but your mental functioning and energy will, as well. This is great news for many people who lose energy as they age.

Reduce Insulin Resistance

Insulin is perhaps the most well-known hormone, as the number of people diagnosed with diabetes only continues to rise. But insulin does not only affect people with diabetes but for everyone. This hormone, produced by the pancreas, is released after eating to allow the cells to absorb and utilize glucose as an energy source. But, often, our sensitivity to insulin decreases as we age or put on weight. The cells can become resistant to insulin, which leads to them being unable to absorb the glucose we have ingested. Over time, this causes a buildup of glucose in the bloodstream and, ultimately, diabetes if it is left untreated.

However, whether you have insulin resistance or already have been diagnosed with type II diabetes, you don't have to allow your condition to worsen. You can treat your insulin resistance directly at the source, and in the process, improve the absorption of glucose by your cells. Many people can lower the severity of their insulin resistance or diabetes, and some are even able to treat it completely.

Multiple controlled studies have found that intermittent fasting can both treat insulin resistance and lower blood glucose levels. Some studies have found that intermittent fasting can even be as effective, if not more effective, than dieting for lowering blood glucose levels.

Reduce Excess and Chronic Inflammation

Inflammation plays an essential role in human health. Without inflammation, we would be the victim of any germ or bacteria that attempted to leave our body. This is why people with a compromised immune system can get sick and pass away so easily.

But, while it might be important to have a functioning immune system that will increase inflammation when we are sick or injured, sometimes we develop excess or chronic inflammation, which is also detrimental to our health. Sadly, cases of excessive and chronic inflammation are becoming more wide-spread due to environmental pollutants, overwork, poor diet, sleep deficiencies, and more. When this happens, the chronic inflammation no longer protects a person from diseases but instead predisposes them to more infection. For instance, studies have found that increased levels of inflammation can lead to heart disease, cancer, rheumatoid arthritis, and much more.

However, you don't have to accept the occurrence of excessive and chronic inflammation helplessly. Studies on the matter have found that intermittent fasting can drastically reduce chronic inflammation levels. One study found that within as little time as a month, participants' inflammation levels were drastically reduced. Another study specifically found that you can achieve these results simply by completing a daily twelve-hour fast for thirty days.

Increase Neural Cells

It is important to take care of brain health as we age, especially as the levels of Alzheimer's disease, Parkinson's disease, and other neurodegenerative diseases are on the rise. But, one way that intermittent fasting can help guard against and treat all brain-related diseases is by increasing the production and repair of neural cells. This is important, as these diseases all cause these vital brain cells to become damaged or stunted overtime.

The result is that if you begin practicing intermittent fasting regularly now, you can reduce your risk of developing a neurological disease in the future. Or, if you already have one, you may be able to reduce symptoms or halt its progression. This is amazing news, as neurological diseases are incredibly hard to treat, even with modern medicine. Studies have specifically shown intermittent fasting to increase cell growth and repair in the cortex, hippocampus, basal forebrain, and nervous system. Along with the decreased risk of disease and disease progression, you can also expect to experience increased mental energy, better focus, improved memory, and a stabilized mood.

Boost Cellular Health

As we age, our cells themselves also age and decrease in age, which is the aging process that we are all so familiar with. But there is a process known as autophagy that can reduce the aging of the cell, and therefore help slightly reduce aging and significantly increase health. There is no method to stop or reverse aging itself, but you can stop and reverse the aging of the cells. The autophagy process causes old, damaged, and dying cells to be replaced with younger and healthier cells, allowing you to maintain health. The process of autophagy is critical for maintaining homeostasis, and if it is malfunctioning, it leads to increased aging and disease.

Researchers have long studied this process, even going to far as to search for drugs that can induce the process of autophagy to treat people with chronic and terminal illnesses. But you can induce autophagy without drug treatments with intermittent fasting. Studies have found that by activating the autophagy process, intermittent fasting can even help your vital stem cells to regenerate themselves.

Lessen Oxidative Stress

Toxins cause oxidative stress. We can develop these toxins when we breathe in poor quality air, don't sleep well, eat poor quality food, apply damaging substances to our skin, and much more. We even develop this oxidative stress when our cells convert fuel to energy, meaning that even if we live in a clean environment, sleep perfectly, and only eat organic food, we would still develop oxidative stress, thereby causing damage to our cells. As our cells develop this damage from oxidative stress, we slowly lose our health and energy, producing an increased risk of disease.

However, studies have shown that intermittent fasting not only increases the rate our cells develop oxidative stress, but it also increases our body's natural antioxidants to fight against this damage directly.

Improve Mental Well-Being

Poor mental health is becoming more common than ever, with over forty-million Americans suffering from one form of mental illness or another, and many others struggling with short-term depression and anxiety. One of the most common causes of disability in middle-aged Americans (as well as those who are young) is chronic severe depression. Yet, a majority of these people never seek professional help.

While I urge you always to seek professional help for your mental health, you can also practice intermittent fasting. Studies have found that with short-term fasting, people can significantly improve their everyday mood, tranquility, alertness, and even the feeling of euphoria. Not only that but also the symptoms of severe depression can be improved with fasting.

250

Treat or Prevent Disease

While we cannot guarantee that intermittent fasting will prevent you from developing a disease or treat an infection you already have, many studies have proven that fasting can help. These studies have shown that fasting a person can menage their symptoms, possibly reverse the condition, and significantly reduce your likelihood of ever developing a disease. Now that we have looked at the general ways in which intermittent fasting can improve your health, let's have a look at some of the specific diseases and conditions you can expect short-term fasting to improve.

Polycystic Ovary Syndrome (PCOS)

One common condition that affects women around the world, and the most prevalent of the endocrine disorders, is polycystic ovary syndrome. Though, you may know of this condition as the abbreviated PCOS. This condition causes a myriad of symptoms, such as fatigue, obesity, menstrual irregularity, infertility, insulin resistance, body hair, and more. These symptoms can only worsen as a woman age and go through menopause. Yet, despite how it affects the lives of so many women, doctors have to pinpoint the cause of this disorder. So far, it is only believed that genetics, insulin resistance, and excessive chronic inflammation can all contribute to the development and progression of this disorder.

While much still needs to be learned about both this disorder and its treatment, controlled scientific studies have revealed that intermittent fasting can greatly improve a person's life with PCOS. These studies have shown that when a woman practices regular short-term fasting paired with healthy nutrition, she can experience an improvement in many symptoms.

251

It is worth mentioning that the ketogenic diet has also been shown to be an especially helpful treatment option for women with PCOS, meaning that when you combine this diet with intermittent fasting, you can expect to improve your symptoms even further. In the studies on the ketogenic diet, it was found that not only did intermittent fasting improve overall symptoms, but previously infertile women were able to conceive.

Non-Alcoholic Fatty Liver Disease

A common condition in people who have developed excessive body fat, especially when located around the abdomen, is non-alcoholic fatty liver disease. The treatment of this disease is frequently weight loss, which, as you are now well aware of intermittent fasting is ideal for. However, the benefits of intermittent fasting for those with this form of liver disease go beyond just weight loss. After all, while it is most common for people with excessive abdomen fat to develop this disease, a person doesn't even have to be overweight to improve it. This disease is caused when fat builds up in the liver, but for some people, fat will build up in this organ even when they are at healthy body weight, making it even harder to treat. Yet, when fatty liver disease is left untreated, it leads to deteriorating health and may also develop into dangerous liver failure, which requires liver transplantation if the person is to survive.

Intermittent fasting can help because it not only helps you to reduce weight and, therefore, the importance of your liver but also because it changes how your body stores its fat. Through studying fatty liver disease, researchers found that individuals who are more prone to storing fat in their liver also have lower levels of a specific protein gene. The good news is that they also found intermittent fasting increases this protein gene, meaning that your liver is less likely to hold onto fat and more likely to shed excess weight. This can help both people who are currently seeking to rid themselves of non-alcoholic fatty liver disease and those who hope to prevent it in the future.

Diabetes

A person who is experiencing severe diabetes and having to undergo insulin treatment may be unable to practice intermittent fasting. Only your doctor will be able to determine whether or not you can safely practice short-term fasting. But, if your condition isn't as severe and your doctor believes it to be safe in your circumstance, then you will be happy to know studies have found intermittent fasting to be incredibly beneficial. Even if you cannot at this time practice intermittent fasting, you may still be able to improve your health enough through the ketogenic diet, at which time you could also take up intermittent fasting under your doctor's discretion.

As you know, intermittent fasting treats excessive weight gain, insulin resistance, and high blood sugar, so it is clear to see why it would help treat diabetes, which is characterized by these three occurrences. Intermittent fasting is so successful that one recent study even found that it was highly effective for type diabetes II patients who were reliant on insulin injections. The participants in this study practiced their fasting closely under their doctor's care multiple times a week. After a short time following their fasting schedule, they were able to completely reverse their insulin resistance, manage blood sugar levels, reduce excess body weight, and even stop their medication.

Alzheimer's Disease

Something that many of us begin to worry about as we age, especially if we have seen relatives go through it in the past, is Alzheimer's disease. This devastating disease not only separates family members in death but also in life. It separates a person from their very understanding and memory of themselves. Sadly, the rate of people with Alzheimer's disease has only continued to skyrocket over the past few decades, with it now being the sixth leading cause of death. The numbers have risen so much that, between the years 2000 and 2015, the rate of people increased by a shocking one-hundred and twenty-three percent, and it is only continuing to rise.

Sadly, science still does not have an answer on how to stop or reverse the disease. However, it has been shown that intermittent fasting can reduce a person's risk of developing it and lessen the severity. A large part of the reason that intermittent fasting is successful is that Alzheimer's disease consists of a mitochondrial cell dysfunction, although it has many other facets as well, such as dysfunctions in the immune system, protein genes, brain cells, and more. When these dysfunctions occur, it causes plaque to buildup in the neurofibrillary of the brain, causing oxidative stress, excessive chronic inflammation, and further mitochondrial dysfunction. It is a vicious cycle where the symptoms continuously cause the disease to worsen, which in turn makes the symptoms also worsen.

The many components of Alzheimer's disease lead to the brain's neurons becoming insulin resistant, and when they are no longer able to absorb the glucose needed, they can also no longer fuel the cells, leading to cellular starvation and death. But as intermittent fasting repairs mitochondrial cells and increases them in number, it can increase the number of cells able to fuel off of non-glucose fuels. It can also treat the insulin resistance itself and cause the production of ketones to fuel the non-mitochondrial neural cells.

Cancer

Lastly, studies have found that intermittent can reduce your likelihood of developing cancer and help make treatment more successful. As you are aware, intermittent fasting can help treat oxidative stress and cellular damage, both of which cause cancer. By reducing this damage, you can thereby reduce your risk of developing cancer in the future.

But that is not all. While human studies still need to be conducted, a study on mice found that when practicing short-term fasting chemotherapy treatment becomes more successful in targeting and treating both breast cancer and skin cancer. Not only did the chemotherapy itself become more effective, but the mice' immune systems also were better able to fight off the cancerous cells and growths, which is essential as chemotherapy is well-known for reducing a person's immune system drastically.

Chapter Three

THE PROS AND CONS OF INTERMITTENT FASTING

There are pros and cons to every lifestyle. For instance, when you are eating a healthy and nutritious diet, you may lose weight and gain health but be unable to eat all your favorite foods in the amount you would like. On the other hand, when you eat junk food all the time you may enjoy yourself, but you will lose health and gain weight. In the same way, there are naturally both pros and cons to intermittent fasting, and by understanding what they are, you can better manage your lifestyle. Like all things, you will find that these pros and cons are most evened out when intermittent fasting is done in moderation. If a person only rarely practices fasting, then they will, in turn, only experience a few of the benefits. On the other hand, if they practice intermittent fasting overly enthusiastically and for longer periods than healthy, then they will experience more of the drawbacks.

Thankfully, with a balanced intermittent fasting schedule, you can find yourself experiencing many of the benefits and few, if any, of the drawbacks. In this chapter, we will be detailing the pros and cons to make it easier for you to make the most of this lifestyle.

While some pros and cons of intermittent fasting are universal, others can be affected by gender and age. In this chapter, we will be exploring what pros and cons you individually may experience as a woman in or over her fifties.

THE POSITIVES OF INTERMITTENT FASTING

1. Boost Weight Loss

Most people discover intermittent fasting either because they want to lose weight or gain health benefits. But, sometimes losing weight can accomplish both of those simultaneously, as a high body fat percentage can increase high blood pressure, cholesterol, and early mortality. Whether you are hoping to gain these health benefits by losing weight or wish to lose weight to feel more comfortable in your skin, you will love the way that intermittent fasting can boost your weight loss.

Many people struggle to find success in typical diets. This is often due to too many crash and fad diets being designed in a way to trigger rapid and quick weight loss, which is unsustainable. The result is either a weight loss plateau or even weight gain over time. But, with intermittent fasting, you can target stubborn weight that won't go anywhere with diets or healthy eating alone.

The human body naturally does better with having specific windows of time for eating, digesting, and burning off fat. But, with our modern society, many people will graze throughout the day, throwing off the natural windows and impeding weight loss and maintenance. The result is that even when a person eats healthfully and exercise, they can still get stuck in weight loss plateaus or gain excess weight.

When we go back to our natural eating and fasting windows, we can begin to experience the real benefits of natural weight loss and maintenance that the human body is designed to accomplish. Not only do fasting periods help to lower your caloric intake, allowing you to lose weight, but it also allows you to still maintain proper eating and nutrition during your eating windows. You can even still enjoy some of your favorite comfort foods in moderation while losing weight!

Controlled scientific studies on intermittent fasting have regularly found that it is more effective than dieting. Researchers have compared the effects of fasting to a multitude of typical diets, and repeatedly intermittent fasting is more effective. This is mostly because not only does intermittent fasting reduce caloric intake naturally and without effort, but also because it increases a person's metabolism. This means that a person is taking in fewer calories while burning more.

2. Balance Important Hormones

One of the most important hormones for our sleep cycles is melatonin. The human body will naturally produce this hormone at night to help us drift off to sleep and stay asleep until morning. But many people still experience sleep disorders. Whether a person has difficulty falling asleep or staying asleep, it will affect their sleep hormones, and their sleep hormones will, in turn, affect their sleep further. This is why a person's sleep disorder will often become more severe over time. As when a person is not sleeping well, their body will no longer produce melatonin properly, and when this happens, the decrease in melatonin will only exacerbate the problem. This disrupts in a person's sleep, and melatonin not only will make them sleepier, but it will also predispose a person to a variety of diseases and weight gain.

Another hormone that will be affected by fasting is cortisol, also known as the stress hormone. When this hormone is increased, not only will a person feel more stressed out and anxious, they will also gain weight more easily, experience increased fatigue, and have trouble falling asleep at night.

Thankfully, studies have found intermittent fasting can help balance a person's cortisol and melioration levels. It does this in a variety of ways. For instance, it can help to reduce cortisol by balancing and regulating blood sugar levels. By balancing cortisol, it sets off a chain reaction that improves the balance of other hormones, including melatonin. One simple change can benefit many hormones and systems within your body.

3. Improve Heart Health

As we age, we all must take even more care of our heart health. After all, heart disease is the number one killer of both men and women. While most often doctors educate men on the symptoms and warning signs of heart attacks, women are often forgotten, leading to increased risk of death. This means women must be extra vigilant, taking care of their heart health and educating themselves on the warning signs of heart attacks.

One crucial way to increase heart health is to watch your cholesterol. There is not a single type of cholesterol, but several. The two main types include LDL, which is known as the "bad" cholesterol, and HDL, known as the "good" cholesterol. While LDL cholesterol will increase your risk of heart attack and heart disease, HDL cholesterol will protect your heart health and remove LDL cholesterol from your body.

Studies on individuals with a high body fat percentage found that when intermittent fasting is practiced, not only is LDL cholesterol lowered, but the number of blood triglycerides is also reduced. It is important to lower these triglycerides, as they are a form of fatty acids that are the building blocks of cholesterol. When we decrease our triglyceride level, it, in effect, makes cholesterol less harmful and reduces our heart health risks.

High blood pressure is a sign of ill heart health, and long-term high blood pressure will increase the damage to your cardiac health and not only increase the risk of heart attack, but also heart disease, stroke, and more. Sadly, many women struggle to lower their high blood pressure, and as a result, are put on medication. Thankfully, studies have found that intermittent fasting can lower blood pressure to a healthy level. This is because when you are fasting, the body will naturally burn its fat and ketones for fuel, and when it is doing this, the liver is unable to produce harmful substances, such as LDL cholesterol, that raise blood pressure.

4. Increase Mental Energy and Efficiency

We all need mental energy to get through the day. When our mind is sluggish, we are unable to think, accomplish anything, and sometimes we may be unable even to stay awake. We have all had troubles at times focusing on work, completing a math problem, remembering what we have read, and so on. This is all due to a lack of mental energy and efficiency. You may think that intermittent fasting would further reduce your mental state, as hunger makes focusing difficult, but the opposite is exact.

Firstly, when done correctly, intermittent fasting reduces hunger, which means that once your body adjusts, you won't have to worry about hunger pangs distracting you. Intermittent fasting can help to improve your mental energy and alertness by increasing your body's natural production of norepinephrine, also known as adrenaline. This natural chemical is an important neurotransmitter within the body, which allows us to increase mental energy, alertness, and efficiency. While further studies on this aspect need to be completed on humans, studies in rats have found that intermittent fasting increases neural cells and connections within the brain. This increase in connections and cells results in a natural increase in mental agility, thought speed, focus, and neural cell communication.

There is an essential hormone within the brain, known as brain-derived neurotrophic factor (BDNF), and studies have proven that intermittent fasting promotes increased levels of this vital hormone. This is important, as when BDNF levels are low, it results in anxiety, depression, and other mental illnesses.

5. Reduce the Potential Risk of Developing Cancer

Of course, nobody can promise that any lifestyle choice will prevent you from developing cancer in the future. However, studies have found that intermittent fasting can potentially reduce your risk. Further studies are ongoing, but current research through animal studies have proven promising. For instance, it was found that rats with tumors survive longer when placed on fasting schedules than the control group.

A human study found that when people practice intermittent fasting while undergoing chemotherapy treatment for cancer, the adverse side effects such as nausea, weakness, and fatigue are reduced. This means that even if a person does develop cancer, intermittent fasting can still help.

Other studies have found that intermittent fasting may reduce the growth of cancer cells and tumors, increasing the patients' likelihood of survival and overcoming cancer.

6. Increase Longevity

Early studies on animals have found that by including intermittent fasting, an animal can experience an increased lifespan. These studies found that even if animals had a higher body fat percentage than the control group, by including intermittent fasting, they were able to increase their lifespan and longevity.

This makes sense, as intermittent fasting has many health benefits, and when all of these benefits are compounded together, it naturally results in a longer lifespan.

7. Lifestyle Ease

We all want improving health and weight, but it is important also to have an easier lifestyle. When it is difficult to gain health and weight, many of us end up failing, as life is already busy and difficult enough without adding added worry and tasks. If a person cook more, eat more frequently, and always worry about a diet, they are unlike to stick to it, as it is merely is unmaintainable.

But intermittent fasting is not a diet, and it results in a much simpler lifestyle. After all, since you have specific fasting windows, it lessens the amount of food you have to cook and how frequently you have to eat, making life easier. The result is that when you are busy, not only do you not have to cook as regularly, but you also don't have to resort to eating junk food, as you can schedule your fasting windows around when you are most busy.

THE POTENTIAL DOWNSIDES OF INTERMITTENT FASTING

1. Getting Started Takes an Adjustment

Any lifestyle change takes an adjustment, and it can take months for something to become a habit. Naturally, intermittent fasting is quite an adjustment for people who are used to grazing on food throughout the day. This means that if you push yourself to go into an advanced version of intermittent fasting when you first begin, you can become overwhelmed. But if you start slowly and allow your body to adjust in its own time, you will find it happens much more naturally and becomes easy to stick to.

You don't have to deprive yourself of food when you are hungry and suffer through hunger pangs. Instead, practice fasting when you are naturally satisfied and eat when you are hungry. If you slowly increase the length of your fasting window, your body will adjust without difficulty, and before long, your body will discover the eating and fasting windows that the human body is naturally inclined to.

2. Potential to Overeat

While intermittent fasting should naturally reduce caloric intake, if a person pushes themselves to fast when they are overly hungry, it might lead to overeating during their eating window. This is because the person feels hungry for so long when fasting when they can finally eat their body believes it must make up for the calories it missed. The result is that the person either hits a weight loss plateau or even experience increased weight.

Thankfully, this is easy to avoid. If you listen to your body by eating when you are hungry and fasting when you are satisfied, you shouldn't overeat. By practicing eating mindfully and slowly, you can also avoid overeating, and you will become more attuned to your body and know when you have eaten enough and can stop.

3. Possible Leptin Imbalance

The hormone leptin is important as it signals to your body that you are full have no longer need to eat. But when a person practices intermittent fasting, it may temporarily disrupt this hormone's production. However, this is usually only a short-term problem, and once a person's body adjusts to their fasting and eating windows, their leptin will balance itself out.

Typically, a leptin imbalance is only a real problem when a person dives head-first into intermittent fasting and attempt to practice advanced level fasting when they are still only a beginner.

4. You May Become Dehydrated

Many people do not drink enough water. In general, doctors recommend that we drink half of our body's weight in pounds in ounces of water. This means that if you weigh two-hundred pounds, you should be drinking one-hundred ounces of water daily.

Not only do many people not drink enough water as it is, but this can make dehydration worse when a person is practicing fasting. This is because fasting boosts the metabolism, and when your cells are in a metabolic accelerated state, they require more water for fuel. If you are not giving them enough water during periods of fasting, you can quickly become dehydrated. Not only that but when fasting, you are likely to lose a lot of water weight, which can result in dehydration and a deficiency in electrolytes. Make sure that you not only drink plenty of water but also consume enough electrolytes to prevent this. Thankfully, dehydration is easy to avoid if you remain proactive.

5. Not Everyone Can Practice Intermittent Fasting

Intermittent fasting is a beautiful and healthy lifestyle for the general population. After all, the human body is designed for practice periods of fasting naturally. However, not every person can practice fasting. Some people, due to chronic illness, may be unable to participate. Ultimately, you must ask your doctor if you are healthy enough to practice short-term fasting.

For instance, people with severe diabetes, metabolic disorders, or those who are pregnant may be unable to practice fasting, even short-term. Whenever you are making a lifestyle change, it is essential first to discuss the matter with your doctor to determine if it is a healthy choice for you individually.

Chapter Four

BUSTING THE MYTHS ABOUT INTERMITTENT FASTING

With the number of fad and crash diets that have come and gone through the ages, there have grown many misconceptions and myths about intermittent fasting. People believe that it is healthier to eat smaller frequent meals, that fasting induces a starvation state, that it will trigger lean muscle loss and more. Thankfully, these myths are simply that: a myth. In this chapter, we will debunk and bust these myths apart with fact and science, so that you can have full confidence in your new lifestyle to gain health and lose weight.

Fasting Induces Starvation

It is commonly believed that fasting induces starvation, which is unhealthy. But this simply is not true. This misconception is understandable, as the fasted state is also referred to as the starved state. However, medically starvation and fasting are very different. While fasting is natural, controlled, and allows a person to consume still all the nutrients and calories their body requires, the same is not true of starvation. Often, fasting is uncontrolled, and it results in a deficiency in nutrients and calories, leaving a person without the vital fuel, vitamins, and minerals their body requires.

People already fast on a nightly basis while asleep, and when you practice intermittent fasting, you do this more purposefully and for

267

slightly longer periods. You still enjoy large, calorie-dense, and healthy meals, along with plenty of fluids throughout the day.

Fasting Causes Lean Muscle Loss

Once again, this fast take root in the false idea that fasting results in deficient nutrient intake. This isn't true! Sure, long-term fasting in which a person is not consuming the nutrients the human body requires, such as in political hunger strikes, might result in lean muscle loss. But the same is not true of healthy short-term fasting. When you practice intermittent fasting, you will be consuming your daily protein requirements during your feeding window, and this protein will stick with you throughout the day for fuel, ensuring you don't lose muscle mass.

Even if you practice a twenty-hour fast, you won't lose muscle mass if you do it properly by consuming plenty of protein and healthy fats during your eating window. Not only will the protein keep your muscles healthy, but the fat will also be transformed into ketones for added fuel, ensuring that your body does not become weakened.

Scientific studies have found that when athletes fast for twelve to twenty hours, there is no risk of muscle loss. Fasting up to forty-eight hours is generally safe (for healthy individuals) as long as a person refuels with the needed nutrients afterward. Although, intermittent fasting is short-term fasting that never goes longer than twenty-four hours. Keep in mind that when you eat a large meal before your fast, that the protein is not all absorbed within a few hours. Instead, protein takes time to be fully absorbed by the body, ensuring that you have protein for fuel all day long. Different sources of protein also absorb at different rates. For instance, the protein within eggs absorbs at a rate of 2.9 grams per hour, whereas a soy protein shake absorbs at a rate of 3.9 grams an hour. If you eat a large meal such as a calorie-rich salad, including chicken, boiled eggs, cheese, bacon, and nuts as protein sources, you will find that you have more than sufficient protein to fuel you throughout your fast.

Humans Can't Survive Without Water

It is a common misconception that you are unable to drink during periods of intermittent fasting. This isn't true! Sure, some religions abstain from all liquids during fasting, such as Muslims during Ramadan. However, this is not a facet of intermittent fasting. Quite the contrary, individuals are encouraged to drink plenty of water to stay hydrated during their fasting window.

Along with water, you can also enjoy calorie-free drinks such as flavored waters, sugar-free sports drinks, tea, and coffee. Artificial sweeteners and sugar alcohols shouldn't be included during your fasting window, though, so no Diet Coke! Why shouldn't these be enjoyed? Because while they may be zero-calorie, your body still has to digest the sweeteners, which will interfere with your fasting. However, you can enjoy stevia leaf extract, which is an herb. This herb is sweet and can be added to drinks, such as coffee and tea.

It is Healthier to Eat Small Frequent Meals

The myth that it's healthier to eat small frequent meals, rather than a few large meals, has no basis in science. This myth began due to unsubstantiated diets that were popular in the '80s and '90s. When you eat smaller frequent meals, your body is always in a fed state where it is forced to digest and absorb the food you have eaten. Your digestive system never gets a chance to rest, and you are rarely able to burn off your body fat. On the other hand, when you go longer periods between your meal, not only does your digestive system get a break from the constant effort of digesting food, you also get an opportunity to burn off your body fat instead of unneeded food.

Once you adjust to intermittent fasting, you shouldn't even feel the need to snack, as your body will learn that you don't have to be putting more calories always. Instead, you will learn to stay satisfied and energized by the nutrients in large meals. Many people believe that eating small, frequent meals boosts your metabolism while large, infrequent meals slow it, but again, this is not true and has no basis in science. This belief mostly began because people misunderstood how the digestive system works. As the body must expend energy to digest a meal, these people believed that by eating frequently, they could harness this use of energy to promote the burning of calories and body fat. Yet, what these people did not understand is that the energy expended during digestion is not affected by how frequently you eat, but rather how many calories you eat. This means that if you eat 12,000 calories in a day, you will expend the same amount of energy to digest them; whether you eat them in small frequent meals or large, infrequent meals, it doesn't change.

Since the frequency of your meals will not affect the number of calories you burn in a day, instead, it is important to limit calorie intake. Intermittent fasting allows you to restrict your calorie intake naturally while you remain satisfied and consume enough nutrients, allowing you to lose weight. You can further compound this benefit by exercising and incorporating the ketogenic diet.

The Brain Will Be Starved of Glucose

The brain requires glucose for fuel, as fatty acids are unable to pass through the blood-brain barrier to fuel your neural cells. However, this does not mean that your brain will be starved while fasting. You don't have to keep ingesting carbohydrates regularly. In fact, out of the three nutrients of protein, carbs, and fat, the only type that humans can live without is carbohydrates. So, how does the brain need glucose, but we also don't need carbs? Simply, the human body is designed in a way that it can survive without a constant carbohydrate/glucose intake. Since glucose is such an important fuel source, the body has its ways to produce this fuel. When a person has burned off all the glucose within their body, then the process of gluconeogenesis will convert amino acids (protein) into the glucose our cells require. Therefore, as long as you eat enough protein, you will always have enough glucose for your brain cells!

Not only will gluconeogenesis ensure you always have enough glucose, but you require less glucose when in a fasted state than when in a fed state. This is because the body will produce ketones when in a fasted state, which can pass through the blood-brain barrier and be used as fuel for the brain. Not only can ketones be used as fuel for the brain, but also for other cells in the body. This is good news, as ketones are a healthier fuel source that reduces the production of free radicals in the body and increase energy levels.

Fasting Results in Binge Eating and Weight Gain

While it is true that a person can binge eat, and therefore gain weight, while practicing intermittent fasting, this is true of any

271

lifestyle. Intermittent fasting does not cause or promote binge eating, and it is entirely dependent on a person's individual choices.

Actually, as many people adjust to intermittent fasting, their overall hunger reduces, as the body realizes, it doesn't need a constant supply of excessive calories. As a person's desire reduces, so too will the amount of food they consume. When you first begin practicing intermittent fasting, you can reduce the risk of binge eating after a fast by slowly and mindfully eating. Instead of sitting in front of the TV or looking at your phone while you eat, slowly enjoy your meal, appreciating each and every bite. Be sure to drink plenty of water, as well!

You can also reduce the likelihood of binge eating by starting your fasting journey slowly. Don't jump right into doing sixteen-hour or twenty-hour fasts. Instead, start with a twelve-hour fast and gradually increase the length of the fast until you naturally reach your quick length goal.

Fasting Reduces Athletic Performance

Athletes commonly worry about lifestyle changes affecting their athletic performance, and for a good reason. But you will be happy to know that when intermittent fasting is done correctly, it won't interfere with your athletic performance. This is especially good for women as they age, as it is important to remain active in promoting healthy aging.

When you first begin practicing fasting, you may be slightly weaker if you push yourself to start too quickly. But, if you start slowly, listening to your body's natural needs, you should find that your energy levels remain intact. But, even if you do feel slightly weaker, this is temporary and will go away once your body adjusts to the change. Once your body adjusts, you won't lose energy as even when in a fasted state, your body will have stores of amino acids, fatty acids, and ketones to burn for fuel. Not only will your body burn off ingested calories, but also body fat, allowing you to lose weight more effectively than when not fasting.

If you do start to feel a reduction in energy, it is more likely due to dehydration or an electrolyte imbalance. Be sure to ingest your daily recommendation of water electrolytes, no matter what. If you suspect you might have an electrolyte imbalance, your doctor can run a simple blood panel to know for sure.

Fasting Can Damage Health

When all your life you have heard fake "science" promoted by crash diets, it's easy to believe that intermittent fasting might harm your health. But the truth is that independent and controlled scientific studies have time and again found short-term fasting not only to be safe but that it also promotes overall health. You can gain a healthier body weight, lower cholesterol, and triglycerides, manage blood sugar, increase energy, and more.

When done as instructed in this book, intermittent fasting does not cause harm to healthy individuals. Although it is important to note that those with certain chronic illnesses and diseases may be unable to handle intermittent fasting, therefore, discuss this lifestyle change with your doctor, and they will be able to evaluate whether or not your health can handle it.

Chapter Five

TRICKS TO SUCCEED WITH INTERMITTENT FASTING

Intermittent fasting is much easier than people first believe, as you pair your fasting periods with feasting periods full of nutritious and satisfying food. Therefore, you stay full during your fasting period, much unlike the meal skipping that most people experience. As long as you start slowly and allow your body to adjust naturally, it should be a simple process. Although, if you do struggle, you should find that after the first five days, things become easier, as after this period, your body will begin to adjust, and fasting will become routine. In this chapter, we will go over some tips and tricks that can make your intermittent fasting journey easier, helping you to gain success, lose weight, and achieve better health.

RESEARCH, RESEARCH, RESEARCH

It's easy to want to jump right into intermittent fasting once you learn of the benefits it has to offer and humanity's history of naturally including fasting in daily life. But if you jump head-first into a new lifestyle without fully understanding it, you are likely to make mistakes that you will later regret. Instead of starting your fasting journey while only halfway through this book, first read each chapter to gain the knowledge and understanding you need to attain success. Research will be your friend, as when you gain experience, you can avoid mistakes and make the journey easier.

UNDERSTAND YOUR MOTIVATION

Making a lifestyle change when only half understanding your motivation is a setting yourself up to quit halfway through. Any lifestyle change takes effort, and if we only have vague ideas of "I want to be healthier" or "I want to weigh less," we can quickly become defeated at the first sign of hurdles. Instead, sit down and write out a list of attainable goals you hope to succeed with. For instance, what aspects of your health do you want to improve? Do you want to lower your cholesterol? Improve your blood pressure? Manage your blood sugar? Reduce daily fatigue? Reduce insomnia to get two more hours of sleep a night? If you want to lose weight, set yourself both short-term and long-term goals. For instance, in the short-term, you can try to lose ten pounds, but maybe long-term, you want to lose fifty.

By having these goals, you will be motivated to overcome the hurdles that come your way, gaining success, and enjoying a better lifestyle.

SLOW AND STEADY WINS THE RACE

When you are excited about succeeding, losing weight, and gaining health, then it is easy to want to rush into intermittent fasting. After you are armed with all the knowledge you need to succeed, you might want to start right off with a 16/8 or even a 20/4 fast. But this is only setting yourself up for failure, just like the hare in the fable "The Tortoise and the Hare." Instead of seeking the fastest way to your goal, find the most successful approach. What does this mean? Don't jump into the more difficult fasting periods. Rather, start with a 12/12 fast or skipping a meal when you aren't hungry. Just be sure that when you do eat that you eat healthy and nutritious food! You can also start by cutting out snacks and training both your mind and body to not eat between mealtimes. After you adjust to these smaller changes, you can slightly increase your fasting window every few days until you reach your desired fasting length.

DRINK PLENTY OF WATER

The importance of staying hydrated cannot be overstated. The truth is that most Americans do not drink their recommended daily intake, which can lead to headaches, migraines, fatigue, stress, false hunger pangs, and more. In fact, by the time you are feeling thirsty, you already are slightly dehydrated. Don't forget to drink your daily intake of water, which is half of your body's weight in pounds in ounces. This means that if you weigh one-hundred and fifty pounds, you should be drinking seventy-five fluid ounces of water, at least, daily.

When you are dehydrated, you can experience false hunger pangs, making you believe that you need to eat when you don't. If you find yourself feeling hungry during your fasting window, before ending your fast early and eating a snack, instead try drinking a glass of water. If you have trouble remembering to drink water, then keep a reusable water bottle at hand at all times and try using a water tracking smartphone app.

AVOID TEMPTATION

While we may not always avoid being around our favorite tempting foods when possible, don't put yourself in a situation to give in to your cravings. For instance, if you know you have a habit of giving in and eating specific junk foods, try not to keep them at home.

But, avoiding temptation is not always about avoiding your favorite foods, but rather timing when you eat them. For instance, if you have a plan to go out to coffee or for drinks with friends, then don't plan your fast during this time. Instead, work your fast around your schedule so that you can enjoy getting food and drinks with friends without impeding your fasting schedule or weight loss. You can still fully enjoy yourself and experience the benefits of intermittent fasting.

You might also consider tailoring where you go out with friends based on the menu. If you are trying to lower your blood sugar, then instead of going out for ice cream, it would be better for your health to find a healthier alternative until your fasting schedule improves your health. Instead of ice cream, you might choose to go out for coffee or get a slightly healthier dessert option, even.

ENJOY THE CAFFEINE BOOST

If you have high blood pressure, you should watch the caffeine, but if you have normal or low blood pressure, you can generally feel free to enjoy a caffeine boost you help you through your fast. Of course, like all medical decisions, you should ask your doctor about your personalized caffeine intake recommendation.

You will find that caffeine can be especially helpful when you are first adjusting to a fasting lifestyle, as it can reduce appetite, helping you to feel more satisfied between meals. Not only that, but it also will provide you with a nice energy boost.

Just remember not to add anything with calories to your coffee during a fasting window, meaning no sugar, cream, or milk. Save these ingredients for your eating windows, instead. If you dislike black coffee or tea, you can add sugar-free natural stevia sweetener during a fasting window. You can also use sugar-free gum to help reduce cravings during the initial adjustment period.

STAY BUSY

It's easy to think that you don't want to stress while busy, and while you may want to avoid changing lifestyles during stressful periods, it is best to take up intermittent fasting when you are working. After all, many people will snack out of boredom, or at the very least, are more likely to notice hunger pangs when they have nothing but time on their hands. On the other hand, if you stay busy with work, chores, or hobbies, you will be able to get through the fasting period seemingly more quickly, with fewer noticeable hunger pangs or temptations to snack.

Remember, a watched pot never boils, and time seems to move most slowly when you are watching the clock. So, if you fast when you are too busy to notice the hours pass by, you will find that before you know it, your fasting window ends, and you can enjoy your next meal. This doesn't mean you need to take up intermittent fasting when your job is keeping you busy, but at the very least, try to find tasks you can delve into at home to pass the time.

LIBERALLY SEASON YOUR FOOD

Surprisingly to many people, by piling on the seasonings during meals in the way of spices, herbs, and vinegar, you can wake up your taste buds, thereby feeling satisfied and full for longer periods. These ingredients also contain very few calories, meaning you can add them liberally to your dishes without adverse effects on your weight.

In Western countries, many people under season their dishes, as you can tell when you compare typical American or British dishes to those from Asia, the Middle East, and other countries throughout the world. Instead of merely cooking fish or chicken with a little salt and pepper, try using a recipe that uses a handful of different spices, herbs, and vinegar so that you can enjoy a genuinely flavorful dish. Not only will these dishes help keep you satisfied, but you will also find that they taste better and are more enjoyable.

PRIORITIZE HIGH-QUALITY AND CONSISTENT SLEEP

Sleep is a vital part of health and well-being, and that includes our health while practicing intermittent fasting. Not only that but by scheduling your fasting schedule to overlap with your sleeping schedule, you can accomplish a longer fasting window without hunger. Without trying, we all already fast overnight between dinner and breakfast, so with a little knowledge of intermittent fasting, you can make better use of this time.

If you are going to be having a particularly long overnight fast, it can help to go to sleep early so that you do not become tempted to get a midnight snack. Although, keep in mind that some people find that an overly large dinner can interrupt their quality of sleep, so find what best works for both your sleep and your fasting schedule. When leading a busy life, or distracted by a good book or TV show, it is easy to neglect sleep. But you mustn't do this, as when you do not sleep properly, it will alter your hormonal balance. As you become sleep deprived, the hormone cortisol will increase, which not only increases stress and impedes sleep but also increases hunger and weight gain. Leptin and ghrelin will also become unbalanced, further increasing hunger and overeating, thereby blocking your progress.

Only by prioritizing consistent and high-quality sleep, you can significantly increase your success in fasting, but also improve your overall health and weight.

TRACK YOUR PROGRESS

While you shouldn't obsess or hyper-focus on your fasting schedule and results, as this can make people overly stressed and self-conscious, it is important to at least track the basics of your progress. This is because it can sometimes feel like we are not making any progress as the scale is not moving, and then you realize you are actually down two jean sizes. The range is not always accurate; what is more important is how fat is positioned on your body.

Therefore, don't only weigh yourself, but also measure your stomach, hips, waist, bust, chest, upper arms, forearms, thighs, and calves. You don't have to worry about tracking these measurements or your weight daily, but at least monitor them once every week or every two weeks. And remember, when you do check your weight and measurements, write it down to keep a record!

By tracking your progress, not only will you be able to recognize your achievement better as you are making it, but you will also come to understand your body and its patterns better.

You can track your progress in a small notebook, journal, yearly planner, or there are even several of helpful smartphone apps created for this purpose.

AVOID FASTING WHEN STRESSED

We all have times in our life when everything seems to be going wrong. Perhaps a loved one is in the hospital, something happened to a beloved family pet, or you are going through a breakup. Generally, these are not good times to begin a new lifestyle. Sure, sometimes you may not be able to avoid it if you need to improve your heart health or blood sugar, but if you can help it, try to begin intermittent fasting when life does feel like a burden. If you do choose to practice fasting during these times, offer yourself kindness and compassion. You can practice shorter fasting windows rather than going for more advanced fasting windows. Allow yourself to have a comforting treat from time to time. If you mess up, forgive yourself.

When making a lifestyle change, you must practice self-kindness if you hope to succeed.

Chapter Six

ENJOYING A BALANCED DIET WITH INTERMITTENT FASTING

E ating a balanced diet is much more than simply eating a salad. This is especially true when you are practicing intermittent fasting, as you need to ensure that you are consuming the proper amount of both macronutrients and micronutrients. But what are these nutrients? Simply macronutrients are the fuel your body consumes in a larger number, including protein, fat, and carbohydrates. On the other hand, micronutrients are equally essential but consumed in a smaller quantity. Micronutrients typically include vitamins, minerals, and phytonutrients found within plants. While a salad may offer you some vegetables, if you don't pair it with plenty of protein and fat, you will be depriving your body of necessary fuel. Not only that, but many people make simple salads with only lettuce, which is low on the nutrition scale. You are much better off consuming a variety of fruits and vegetables to absorb all the micronutrients your body requires. In this chapter, we will examine how you can enjoy a healthy and balanced diet with intermittent fasting.

Salads are a go-to choice for many dieters because they are low in calories and contain vegetables. However, when you are practicing intermittent fasting, you must ensure you consume all the calories and nutrients your body requires during your feeding window, and a simple romaine salad with ranch dressing will not do that. Yet, all salads are not created equal. For instance, you may choose to eat a roasted chicken thigh with a kale salad topped with roasted beets, fresh avocado, toasted almonds, goat cheese, apple, and a rich olive oil vinaigrette. If you make a meal such as this, you will be consuming plenty of protein, healthy fats, and a variety of essential fruits and vegetables. Not only will this meal provide you with the macronutrients and micronutrients your body requires, but it will also leave you full and satisfied for hours to come.

Remember: Don't focus on low-calorie food, but rather nutrient-dense and satisfying meals. This applies whether you are on a standard healthy diet, or if you are pairing the ketogenic diet with intermittent fasting.

Not only do fruits and vegetables offer you a variety of micronutrients that the body requires, but meat can be quite nutritious, as well! While it is important to enjoy red meat in moderation, it has such a high degree of vitamins and minerals that the occasional serving can be incredibly beneficial. Beef is a prime example of nutritious red meat. Beef consists of twenty-six percent protein, which means that for every one-hundred grams of meat you eat, you can get twenty-six grams of vital protein and amino acids to fuel your body throughout your fast. On average, a serving of beef is considered three ounces of meat, which contains twenty-two grams of protein in total. While beef may contain saturated fats, which should be consumed in moderation, it also has other important and healthy fats such as oleic acid, which is commonly found in avocados and olives, palmitic acid, and stearic acid.

The micronutrients in beef, meaning vitamins and minerals, are essential for the human body. However, many of these nutrients are not well absorbed from plant-based sources. We may absorb a small number of the vitamins and minerals we eat from a salad or roasted vegetables, but the human body absorbs these mispronunciations much more effectively from meat. Let's have a look at some of the micronutrients found in large number within beef:

- **Vitamin B12**
  B vitamins are essential for human health, including vitamin B12. This vitamin helps manage our nervous system, neural health, and is used in the formation of blood. But, unlike some of the other B vitamins, B12 can only be found in animal-derived ingredients, such as meat.

- **Vitamin B6**
  Humans need vitamin B6 in larger quantities than some of the other B vitamins, as it plays an important role in the formation of blood. Without enough B6, we become anemic.

- **Iron**
  There are two different types of iron, and it is very important to consume these to prevent anemia. The first type is non-heme iron, which is found in plant-based ingredients. When you consume non-heme iron in plants such as spinach, your system is unable to absorb and make use of a large portion of the iron, making most of it go to waste. On the other hand, meat, such as beef, contains heme iron, which is easily absorbed and utilized by the body. Some people, no matter how much plant-based non-heme iron they consume, will remain anemic and require heme iron from meat to prevent this condition.

- **Selenium**
  Humans only need a small amount of selenium in their diets, but it is hard to come by. Without enough selenium, our metabolism, thyroid function, and immune system all suffer. Thankfully, with beef, you can ensure you are consuming enough selenium without absorbing too much, as can happen with some other sources of selenium.

- **Zinc**
  An essential micronutrient for the immune system, zinc keeps us healthy by fighting off germs such as those that cause the flu and everyday cold. Often, when a person experiences a large number of viral infections, it is due to insufficient consumption of zinc. While there may be supplements on the market of zinc to help you when you come down with a cold, the human body better absorbs this mineral when you consume it in your everyday diet, such as in beef. Not only that, but you will also find it more useful to consume adequate levels of zinc regularly than only when you are sick. This way, it can help prevent you from coming down with illnesses in the first place.

- **Creatine**
  A vital antioxidant, creatine helps us to maintain muscle health, maintain bone density, improve neural functioning, and increase the functioning of our inner organs. Creatine can also increase energy levels, meaning it can help boost your energy when you are adjusting to the intermittent fasting lifestyle.

- **Taurine**
  This nutrient is commonly found within both meat and fish, and it is important for heart and blood health, which

is especially helpful for women as they age. Studies have found that taurine can be especially helpful in the treatment of congestive heart failure, cystic fibrosis, and other heart and blood-related illnesses.

- **Niacin**
  Also known as vitamin B3, niacin is used throughout the human body for basic functioning. Put simply, without niacin, humans could not survive. But this is good news, as by consuming foods rich in niacin such as beef, chicken, salmon, and tuna fish, you can improve many aspects of your health. Niacin is primarily known to help manage heart and brain health, which are two of the most important aspects to focus on as we age.

- **Glutathione**
  One of the most powerful antioxidants known is glutathione. While this antioxidant can often be found in the peel on grapes and wine, one of the most under-rated sources of glutathione is meat. While you can benefit from this antioxidant in any source of beef, you will find that grass-fed beef contains the highest levels of this nutrient and others.

As you can see, there are many reasons to consume meat, as it has many nutrients. Beef is just one prime example. Other meats, such as fish, also offer several micronutrients while having less saturated fats that can raise cholesterol. When consuming fish, the best sources are smaller fish high in fat. The fat in fish is high in omega-3 fatty acids, which most people in Western countries do not consume enough of. This is detrimental, as when we consume low levels of omega-3 and high levels of omega-6 fats, it causes inflammation and increases the risk of disease. But, by lowering your omega-6 intake and increasing your omega-3 consumption, you can greatly improve your health. Fatty fish such as salmon and sardines are two of your best options.

Try to avoid larger fish options, such as tuna, as the larger a fish, the higher mercury contamination it contains. This is because larger fish eat smaller fish, thereby increasing their mercury contents, and when you eat these fish, the mercury contamination crosses over to you. Sardines are one of the best options, as they are rich in omega-3 fatty acids, and since they are small, they contain very little mercury. Sardines are also inexpensive and sold in tin cans, making them stay shelf-stable for long periods. If you purchase bone-in sardines, you can also benefit from an increase in calcium for bone health.

As you can see, both meat and fish have many health benefits. Healthy eating goes beyond eating just fruits and vegetables, but it is about everything you eat. To eat a balanced diet is important to choose a balance of healthy proteins, fats, and carbohydrates. Of course, you do not need to consume many carbohydrates, as this is the one fuel source the body does not require through consumption. The ketogenic diet, which is extremely low carb, can further increase the health benefits you receive through intermittent fasting and boost weight loss. The ketogenic diet can also make intermittent fasting easier, and it prioritizes protein and fat consumption and increases the production of ketones.

When possible, try to choose grass-fed and organic ingredient options, as these not only don't contain harmful substances, they also provide more nutrition. For instance, studies have found that grass-fed butter contains an average of five times the nutrients of grain-fed butter. This increase of nutrients carries over to everything you eat, whether animal-based or plant-based.

It is okay if you can't afford to buy all your ingredients organic and grass-fed, but when you are able, it is best to budget some of your ingredients to at least be higher quality. The best foods to prioritize as organic and grass-fed include meat and vegetables and fruits on the dirty dozen list. The dirty dozen list is fruits and vegetables that contain the highest level of contamination from harmful substances, and therefore are safest to buy organic. This list includes:

- Strawberries
- Spinach
- Nectarines
- Apples
- Peaches
- Pears
- Cherries
- Grapes
- Celery
- Tomatoes
- Sweet bell peppers
- Potatoes

While the ketogenic diet pairs well with intermittent fasting, not everyone chooses to combine the two lifestyles, and that is okay. If you decide to not go on the ketogenic diet, then be sure to prioritize the quality of the carbohydrates you are consuming, as well. You don't want to eat tons of fruit, which is high in glucose and fructose. Fruit is good in moderation, but remember that sugar is sugar, whether it is coming from fruit or cane sugar.

It is best also to choose whole grains rather than processed grains, as the fiber content is higher. This is important, as fiber improves digestive health, allows your body to absorb nutrients better, removes harmful cholesterol from the body, and helps you to remain full and satisfied for longer periods. On the other hand, processed grains that have had most of their fiber removed will spike your blood sugar and in turn, cause a blood sugar crash, making you feel hungry and tired.

When choosing sources of fat, remember that not all fat is created equal. You should prioritize monounsaturated fats such as those in olives, avocados, and nuts. These are the healthiest sources of fats. The second-best source of fat is polyunsaturated fats, which you can find in seeds, walnuts, fish, safflower oil, and soy-based products. The saturated fats found in meats and coconut oil can raise cholesterol, and therefore should be eaten in moderation. Yes, you can enjoy beef and other meats as they have nutritional benefits, but remember always to prioritize the healthier fats over saturated fats. For instance, instead of eating full-fat meat, you may purchase a lower-fat cut off percentage of ground beef and alternatively add fat to your meal with olive oil, avocado oil, or toasted nuts. This will ensure you can both get the nutrients in meat while also prioritizing the best sources of heart-healthy fat.

Chapter Seven

PAIRING INTERMITTENT FASTING WITH THE KETOGENIC DIET FOR THE ULTIMATE LIFESTYLE

Intermittent fasting can be taken to the next level when you pair it with the ketogenic diet. But what is the ketogenic diet? It is a method of eating developed by doctors and researchers a century ago to treat neurological health conditions, such as epilepsy. Over the decades, the method has been improved upon and undergone countless studies. These studies have found that not only does the ketogenic diet improve neurological health, but it also helps heart health, increases weight loss, and more.

The ketogenic diet is a method in which a person consumes very few carbohydrates (on average, twenty-five or fewer net grams a day) and instead prioritizes the consumption of healthy protein and fats. Due to limiting carbs while increasing fats, the ketogenic diet triggers the body to produce ketones as a fourth fuel source. Ketones are also produced when a person practices fasting. This means that when you practice the ketogenic diet, you will already be producing ketones on a constant basis, allowing your body to stay energized and full the entire time you are fasting, as your body is already used to utilizing this energy source. In this chapter, we will explore how you can benefit from pairing the ketogenic diet with intermittent fasting if you so choose.

When the human body is in a fasted state, the mitochondrial cells, with the mitochondria being the powerhouse of the cell, begin to produce ketones. These are a fuel source that, unlike fat, can cross the blood-brain barrier to fuel the neurons in the absence of glucose. But, not only are these ketones produced during a fasted state, but also on the ketogenic diet as the mitochondrial cells will begin producing them upon realizing that your diet is low in carbohydrate and, therefore, glucose.

While the ketogenic diet and fasting have some benefits unique unto themselves, they also share some of the same benefits. Because of this, when you combine the ketogenic diet and intermittent fasting, you can compound upon the benefits for even greater success. For instance, you can expect to experience healthier cholesterol and blood sugar levels sooner than you would by using either the ketogenic diet or intermittent fasting along. Of course, you can also expect to lose weight more quickly, as well.

Many people pair the ketogenic diet and intermittent fasting together, as the high fat and protein contents on the ketogenic diet are ideal to stay full, satisfied, and energized during long periods of fasting. Plus, with the absence of carbohydrates, you won't have to struggle with blood sugar highs and lows during your fasting window. When practiced alone, both the ketogenic diet and intermittent fasting are powerful but paired together; they are an amazing and unstoppable powerhouse.

While you may be able to enjoy foods such as whole-grains, beans, and fruits while you are solely practicing intermittent fasting, this will change if you combine fasting with the ketogenic diet. As you will be eating so few carbohydrates in a day, you will be avoiding grains, beans and legumes, high-starch vegetables, and most fruits. There are a few fruits that can be enjoyed in moderation, such as berries, but most fruits are overly high in sugar. Along with avoiding any carb-heavy ingredients, you will also want to avoid unhealthy fats and instead prioritize the consumption of healthy fats. Remember, since the ketogenic is high in fat, if you eat a large number of unhealthy fats, you can expect it to be detrimental to your health, just as it negatively affects your health when you eat sugary and fried foods. So, instead of eating anything that has a high-fat content, instead choose healthy monounsaturated and polyunsaturated fats in general, with saturated fats from dairy, meat, and coconut in moderation.

When on the ketogenic diet, it is important to keep in mind that there are two types of carbohydrates that you will be calculating: total carbs and net carbs. As you read a nutritional label of a given ingredient, you will always see the total carb count, and sometimes it might even list the net carb count. While you can typically only eat twenty-five carbs on the ketogenic diet, this is a net carb limitation, not a total carb one. But the good news is that even if a nutrition label doesn't list the net carbs, you can easily calculate it yourself!

So, what is the difference between total and net carbs? Net carbs have removed the calculation for any carbohydrates that are not processed by the body and, therefore, won't affect your blood sugar. Most of the time, this calculation removes fiber, but it can also remove sugar alcohols.

As the body does not digest fiber, it will not affect your blood sugar, insulin, or calorie consumption. But fiber is still a form of carbohydrate, which is why it is included in the total carb calculation. Sugar alcohols are a natural sweetener, that much like fiber, are not processed by the body. During the process of digestion, the body is unable to digest sugar alcohols and, therefore, will excrete them, ensuring they don't alter your blood sugar, either. This is why many natural sweeteners, such as Truvia and Swerve, are calorie-free.

If you were to calculate the net carbs in a single serving of strawberries, you would look at the total carb count, which is eleven, and then the dietary fiber count, which is three. When you remove the fiber count from the total carb count, you are left with the net carb count: eight.

You will find that there are many keto-friendly products on the market that use sugar alcohols such as erythritol and xylitol as sweeteners. Along with these two sugar alcohols, the products might also contain stevia leaf extract and monk fruit extract, both of which are also keto-safe. Often, these products will contain the calculated net carb count making it easy on the consumer, as they are marketed to those on a low-carb diet.

The amount of protein a person needs on the ketogenic diet varies based on their body type, activity level, and gender. But, in general, the ketogenic diet focuses on moderate protein consumption, with it making up an average of twenty to twenty-five percent of your diet. Some people may boost their protein intake up even further, to thirty percent, if they are interested in weightlifting and muscle building. It is important to consume adequate protein; otherwise, you will experience lean muscle loss, a weakened immune system, and be at a higher risk of developing common diseases. Thankfully, it is easy to consume enough protein in your daily diet between enjoying meat, fish and seafood, dairy, seeds, nuts, tofu, and eggs.

To know exactly how much you should be eating of the macronutrients (carbs, protein, and fat), you should be eating on the ketogenic diet. You should calculate your macros. Thankfully, this is made easy with online keto calculators. You can find an array of these online calculators online, but the ones from Ruled. Me and Perfect Keto are both good. There are also keto smartphone apps that not only include macronutrient calculators but also easy methods to track your calorie and macronutrient consumption over the day to make it easy to stick to your macros.

Speaking of tracking your macronutrient and calorie consumption, this is generally really important on the ketogenic diet. This is because it is much easier to consume twenty-five net carbs than you might think, and if you aren't tracking your carb intake, you are likely to double or more what you should be eating.

On the ketogenic diet, you can enjoy plenty of healthy fats, fish, seafood, meat, low-starch vegetables, berries, nuts, and seeds. But, to gain the most success, it is better to go into detail about the ingredients you shouldn't be eating. These ingredients can mess up your macronutrient ratio and throw off your nutrition.

FOODS TO AVOID

Grains

While grains may have their health benefits and be full of fiber, you can also get these nutrients elsewhere. The human diet does not require grain consumption. The truth is while grains may have some benefits, they are ridiculously high in both total and net carbohydrates, making them incompatible with the ketogenic diet. A single serving of brown rice contains a shocking forty-two net carbs, which is almost double your net carb intake for an entire day.

Although, some people do try what is known as the targeted ketogenic diet, which is a version of the diet specifically designed for those who complete extended and strenuous workouts. With the targeted ketogenic diet, a person will consume a small serving of a carb-heavy food, such as grains, thirty to forty minutes before working out.

Starchy Vegetables and Legumes

Some vegetables are high in carbohydrates. This includes potatoes, beans, beets, corn, and more. Yes, these vegetables may have nutritional benefits, but you can get these same nutrients in low-carb vegetable alternatives. To put into perspective how high in carbs these options can be, a medium-sized white potato contains forty-three net carbs (more than a serving of brown rice!), a standard sweet potato contains twenty-three net carbs, and a serving of black beans contains twenty-five net carbs.

Better Alternatives:

- Peppers
- Kale
- Radishes
- Cauliflower
- Green beans
- Asparagus
- Spinach
- Avocados
- Zucchini

- Tomatoes
- Celery
- Lettuce
- Swiss chard
- Cucumber
- Cabbage
- Broccoli
- Olives
- Mustard and turnip greens
- Squash

Sugary Fruits

Most fruits contain a high sugar content, meaning that they are also high in carbohydrates, will spike your blood sugar, and cause an insulin reaction. To avoid this, it is important to avoid most fruits. The exception is that you can enjoy berries, lemons, and limes in moderation. Some people will also enjoy a small serving of melon as a treat from time to time, but watch your portion size as it can add up quickly!

Milk and Low-Fat Dairy Products

As you can enjoy dairy products such as cheese on the ketogenic diet, you may consider trying milk. Sadly, milk is much higher in carbohydrates than cheese, with a glass of two-percent milk containing twelve carbs, half of your daily total. Instead, choose low-carb and dairy-free milk alternatives such as almond, coconut, and soy milk.

You may consider using low-fat cheeses instead of full fat to reduce the saturated fats you are consuming. But, if you are looking to reduce your saturated fat intake, choose lighter cuts of meat rather than low-fat dairy products. The reason for this is because when the cheese is made with low-fat dairy, it naturally has a higher carbohydrate content, which will cut into your daily net carb total.

Cashews, Pistachios, and Chestnuts

While you can enjoy nuts and seeds in moderation, keep in mind that nuts contain a moderate level of carbohydrates, and therefore should be eaten in moderation. However, some nuts are high in carbs and thus are not fed on the ketogenic diet, including cashews, pistachios, and chestnuts.

If you want to enjoy nuts, instead of these options, you can fully enjoy almonds, pecans, walnuts, macadamia nuts, and other options.

Most Natural Sweeteners

While you can certainly enjoy sugar-free natural sweeteners such as stevia, monk fruit, and sugar alcohols, you should avoid natural sweeteners that contain sugar. Suffice to say the sugar content makes these sweeteners naturally high in carbs. But, not only that, they will also spike your blood sugar and insulin. This means you should avoid things such as honey, agave, maple, coconut palm sugar, and dates.

Alcohol

Alcohol is not generally enjoyed on the ketogenic diet, as your body will be unable to burn off calories while your liver attempts to process alcohol. Many people also find that when they are in a state of ketosis, they get drunk more quickly and experience more severe hangovers. Not only that, but alcohol adds unnecessary calories and carbohydrates to your diet.

The worst offenders to choose would be margaritas, piña coladas, sangrias, Bloody Mary, whiskey sours, cosmopolitans, and regular beers.

But, if you do choose to drink alcohol regardless of drink in moderation and choose low-carb versions such as rum, vodka, tequila, whiskey, and gin. The next-best options would be dry wines and light beers.

Chapter Eight

HOW TO EXERCISE WHILE FASTING

Frequently, people are told to exercise and decrease calories when trying to lose weight. Simply take in fewer calories and expend more. But, losing weight is not this simple. After all, many people will try this method for years with little to no success in weight loss. That's because while this approach may seem rather simple, there is some important understanding many people are lacking. If you attempt to push yourself through dieting and intense exercise continuously, you will only deprive your body of essential nutrients and wear yourself out both physically and mentally.

Part of the problem that many people run into without realizing is a hormone imbalance. When a person decreases their food intake and increases their exercise in the wrong way, it will cause the hormones cortisol, leptin, and ghrelin to increase. When this happens, a person experiences increased hunger, increased weight retention, and added physical fatigue. Not only do all of these cause problems on their own, but it can also result in a person giving in to cravings and giving up on exercise.

Thankfully, intermittent fasting has been proven through study after study to be much more useful than dieting in weight loss. However, you can further increase weight loss by adding exercise to your routine, as well. In this chapter, you will learn how to pair exercise with intermittent fasting for optimal success, and without creating roadblocks, such as hemorrhage imbalances, that will impede your results.

You will be happy to know that the effects of exercise are increased when you are in a fasted state. This is because you will have few calories in your system. Therefore, your body will be forced to rely on burning off body fat for energy. Studies have repeatedly shown that when a person exercises in a fasted state, they burn off more body fat than they otherwise would. This means you can work out less and experience more weight loss! But, while the idea of increased weight loss may cause you to push yourself more to get the results you hope for sooner, it is important to take your time and listen to your body. If you push your body's limits too much, you can develop not only injuries but also hormonal imbalances and weakened health.

Most people who accomplish low to moderate intensity exercises will not experience diminished athletic performance. However, athletes and those who perform high-intensity exercise might notice a slight decrease in their performance, so they might want to participate in sporting activities during their eating window rather than their fasting window to increase energy.

The reason that athletes and those who practice high-intensity exercises may experience slight performance decreases during their fasting window is due to API energy. This source of energy is a result of glucose being stored within the muscles, which allows people to quickly react at high intensities. For instance, it is API energy that will fuel your body if you suddenly have to begin sprinting from danger. As the glucose for API energy is being stored in your muscles at all times, up to two-thousand calories worth at a time, your muscles can quickly jump to action without preparation. But, if you are in a fasting window without glucose being stored in your muscles, you will find that this energy source is lacking, thereby making short-term/high-intensity exercise more difficult. The result is that those who complete sports, bodybuilding, and CrossFit will be affected.

While you can perform high-intensity exercises while in a fasted state, you must do it while carefully listening to your body, and if you find that you become overly weak, dizzy, or light-headed, then it is important that you either reduce your pace or take a short break before resuming your workout.

You are less likely to notice this decrease in energy if you are only a few hours into your fasting window, but if you are twelve hours or more into a fast, then you are more likely to experience this performance decrease. Therefore, if you do want to practice a high-intensity workout during your fast, try to schedule it earlier in your fasting window rather than later.

If you are not on the ketogenic diet, then it can be a good idea to increase your healthy carbohydrate intake before beginning your fasting window if you plan to exercise. Simply eating some brown rice or starchy vegetables can help you to increase your ATP energy supply, helping you later in the day during your workout.

Thankfully, studies on short-term fasting and exercise have found that as a person adjusts to both fasting and working out, it becomes easier. Over time, your body will adapt to the decreased ATP energy and be able to perform better even when in a fasted state.

The good news for people who don't care for intense exercise is that moderate cardio is the ideal workout for a fasted state. This is because cardio does not use API energy, meaning that you will be able to complete it at full performance without any problems. Many types of exercises can be achieved with cardio, and the weight loss effects of all of them will be increased when you are in a fasted state. This can be especially helpful for women as they age, as cardio improves both heart and lung health.

If you are on the ketogenic diet, then you will be happy to know that cardio doesn't require you to consume a larger quantity of carbohydrates, as it doesn't utilize API energy. You can maintain your state of ketosis and promote weight loss simultaneously. Cardio is especially perfect for completing during your fasting window, as you never want to achieve a cardio workout on a full stomach. While some people may mistakenly eat directly before a cardio workout, this is damaging as the blood flow to your muscles will interfere with your digestive system. When this happens, it can not only cause digestive distress, but it also prevents your body from absorbing the nutrients from your meal. If you are going to be workout out, only do so after fasting for three to four hours minimum.

While many people have been advised by trainers or workout enthusiasts to eat a lot of protein directly before their workout, often in the form of a protein shake or smoothie, new scientific research found that this is not needed. Not only is it doing your body a disservice to eat directly before working out, but studies have found that it does not improve your workout at all. It doesn't even improve bodybuilding, as you can increase muscle growth as long as you eat protein within a few hours of weightlifting.

How you eat and fast can also affect your insulin sensitivity, which is important as reduced insulin sensitivity is a part of and precursor to type II diabetes, which many women develop as they age. In one study, athletes and bodybuilders completed a variety of fasting and eating methods to compare their insulin sensitivity. One group consumed a carb-heavy meal directly before their workout, one trained while in a fasted state, and the control group did not work out at all. All three groups consumed the same meals, and the only thing that varied was when they ate in relation to their workout. The study revealed that while the first and second group ate the same foods and the same amount of food, the group that exercised while in a fasted state experienced improved insulin sensitivity. Not only that, but this group also was able to tolerate glucose better.

The human growth hormone, also known as HGH, experienced increased production when you are in a fasted state. This is good news, as it can help you increase muscle strength and mass while workout out. Even if you are not looking to increase overall muscle mass, we can all benefit from strengthening muscles, especially as they begin to weaken as we age. You can keep your muscles stronger and younger as you age if you practice exercise in a fasted state, at a much more effective rate than if you exercised without fasting. This is important, as when muscles become weakened and aged a person experiences an increased risk of energy, they are more likely to fall, and the body overall begins to run less efficiently.

Pairing exercise and fasting can create antioxidants that reduce fatigue, increase healing, produce more energy, and improve overall health as you age. As you are most likely well aware of, antioxidants are vital for reducing cellular aging and decay. Not only will this protect your muscle health, but overall body health, even the health of your brain.

There are a few things you should keep in mind while working out during a fasted state to get the most out of your workout while saving your energy and maintaining your health. Thankfully, you working out in a fasted state is much easier than you might think, and you will find it much more effective than exercise alone. First, it is often easiest for most people to practice a moderate-range fast of fourteen or sixteen hours, skipping breakfast and making lunch the first meal of the day. If you are doing this, then you can easily workout first thing in the morning when you are a decent way into your fast, and it will be the most productive. You will feel more energy at this time as you are well-rested, and then you can recharge at lunchtime with your meal breaking your fast.

When exercising in this way, your body in a fasted state will activate the sympathetic nervous system, therefore allowing you to burn more fat and lose more weight. But it is important to remember that just because you are fasting doesn't mean you need water any less. It is even more important to stay hydrated. Be sure that while you are exercising, you drink plenty of water and that during your eating window, you consume plenty of electrolytes. Although, you can also purchase zero-calorie sugar-free sports drinks that are naturally sweetened with stevia leaf, and you can enjoy these during even a fasted workout.

When you are exercising, listen to your body and use common sense to know your limits. These limits will vary for everyone based on their exact age, fitness level, health, how long they have been in a fasted state, whether or not they are taking medicine, and more. Only you and your doctor can determine exactly where your limit is, and to avoid pushing past this limit. It is important to listen to all the signs and signals your body is giving you.

If you find that you struggle to exercise after long periods of fasting, then instead do your workout only a few hours into your fast rather than near the end of it. You might find that certain types of exercise are easier for you to complete in a fasted state than others. Or, you might find that there is a specific amount of time after your workout that you feel best eating at. For instance, while one person may be able to wait hours after their workout to eat, another person may only be able to wait thirty to sixty minutes.

Listen to your body and plan your meals, fasting, and exercise routine accordingly.

Chapter Nine

RECIPES

While you can consume any diet while practicing intermittent fasting, you must consume nutritious and healthy foods if you hope to benefit your health. In this chapter, we will share some of our favorite recipes that are full of nutrients necessary in a healthy lifestyle. Some of these recipes will be low-carb/ketogenic, whereas others, so that both individuals who choose to pair the ketogenic diet with fasting and those that do not can equally experience benefits from these recipes.

BREAKFAST

These recipes are the perfect breakfast. Whether you are enjoying breakfast at 7 am or noon, it doesn't matter. You will find that these recipes are not only full of delicious flavor that will bring you back for more time, and again, they are also full of nutrition that will keep you satisfied and healthy.

SWEET POTATO AND CHICKPEA HASH

This hash is simple to cook, but full of flavor and crispy! Not only that, but it is also vegan! Enjoy it served as-is, or you can enjoy it with either freshly sliced avocado or a fried egg for added flavor and nutrition. With this hash, you will stay full and satisfied all day long.

Details:

Number of Servings: **4**

Time Needed to Prepare: 10 minutes
Time Required to Cook: 45 minutes
Total Preparation/Cook Time: 55 minutes

Number of Calories in Individual Servings: 343

Protein Grams: 12
Fat Grams: 17
Total Carbohydrates Grams: 40
Net Carbohydrates Grams: 25

Ingredients:

- Sweet potatoes, cut into 3/4-inch cubes – 1.5 pounds
- Chickpeas, canned, drained and rinsed – 15 ounces
- Bell pepper, red or orange, diced – 1
- Bell pepper, green, diced – 1
- Onion, medium, diced – 1
- Garlic powder – 1 teaspoon

- Sea salt – 1.5 teaspoons
- Olive oil – 2 tablespoons
- Black pepper, ground - .25 teaspoons
- Tahini paste – 4 tablespoons
- Water – 4 tablespoons
- Sea salt - .5 teaspoon
- Lemon juice – 2 tablespoons
- Sriracha sauce – 2 tablespoons

Instructions:

Begin by setting your oven to a temperature of Fahrenheit four-hundred and twenty-five degrees. Then, line a large aluminum baking sheet with either kitchen parchment or a silicone mat.

Place the diced onion, sweet potatoes, and bell peppers on the prepared baking sheet, along with the rinsed chickpeas. Drizzle the olive oil, black ground pepper, garlic powder, and 1.5 teaspoons of sea salt over the vegetables and then toss them all together until the vegetables are well coated in the oil and seasoning.

Spread the vegetable mixture out evenly on the pan so that the sweet potatoes, beans, peppers, and onions are all in a single layer. This will allow the hash to cook consistently and become crispy.

Place the sheet of vegetables in the center of your oven and let it cook for twenty-five minutes, stirring the vegetables once halfway through the cooking time.

Increase the temperature of your oven to Fahrenheit five-hundred degrees, stir the vegetables again, and cook for an additional twenty minutes. Once again, halfway through the cooking time, stir the vegetables.

While the vegetables cook whisk together the tahini paste, water, sriracha sauce, lemon juice, and remaining sea salt.

Once the hash is finished cooking, serve it with the sriracha tahini sauce, and enjoy. Optionally, you can add avocado slices or a fried egg on the side.

OATMEAL PANCAKES

The bananas and oats pair beautifully for a sweet and nutty flavor, but they also add extra value to these pancakes. Rather than making traditional pancakes that contain only refined sugar and flours, you can gain the fiber and nutrients from both the oats and the bananas. These nutrients will keep you healthy and full.

Details:

Number of Servings: **5**

Time Needed to Prepare: 3 minutes
Time Required to Cook: 10 minutes
Total Preparation/Cook Time: 13 minutes

Number of Calories in Individual Servings: 362
Protein Grams: 14
Fat Grams: 6
Total Carbohydrates Grams: 65
Net Carbohydrates Grams: 56

Ingredients:

- Bananas, ripe, large – 2
- Rolled oats – 2.25 cups
- Coconut milk – 1 cup
- Egg – 1
- Maple syrup – 1 tablespoon
- Baking powder – 1.5 teaspoons
- Sea salt - .25 teaspoon
- Cinnamon, ground - .5 teaspoon

- Vanilla extract – 1 teaspoon
- Butter for cooking

Instructions:

Place all of the ingredients, except for the butter, in a blender. Blend on high speed until the oats and bananas have broken down, about one to two minutes.

Heat a large electric griddle or a non-stick skillet over medium-low heat.

Once the griddle or skillet is preheated, add a little of the butter and coat the pan with it. Then, using a small ladle, pour small scoops onto the griddle, with each pancake holding about .25 cups of batter.

Cook the pancakes for two to three minutes before flipping and cooking a couple more minutes.

Serve the pancakes with sliced bananas and maple syrup.

KETO BURRITO WRAP WITH BACON AND AVOCADO

These keto burritos are low in carbs and high in important healthy fats, such as those from avocados. Whether you are on the ketogenic diet or not, you will find that these breakfast burritos are delicious and a great way to start your day! The fats and protein within these burritos will keep you energized and satisfied for hours to come.

Details:

Number of Servings: **2**

Number of Calories in Individual Servings: 426
Protein Grams: 13
Fat Grams: 39
Total Carbohydrates Grams: 6
Net Carbohydrates Grams: 2

Ingredients:

- Eggs – 2
- Bacon, cooked – 4 slices
- Half n' half – 2 tablespoons
- Sea salt - .25 teaspoon
- Black pepper, ground - .125 teaspoon
- Mayonnaise – 2 tablespoons
- Butter – 2 tablespoons
- Roma tomato, sliced – 1
- Romaine lettuce, chopped – 1 cup

- Avocado, sliced - .5

Instructions:

Vigorously whisk together the eggs with the sea salt, black ground pepper, and half n' half until the egg white proteins break down and combine thoroughly with the egg yolk.

In a non-stick skillet over a preheated temperature of medium heat, melt half of the butter. Once the butter has melted, add in half of the egg mixture. Tilt the pan around to ensure the egg covers the entire surface evenly.

Cover the pan with a lid and allow the egg to cook for a minute until set. Once the bottom of the egg is cooked and can move around the pan gently flip it over to cook the other side the rest of the way.

Once both sides of the egg are cooked gently, remove it from the pan and allow it to rest on a plate with a paper towel, allowing it to remove any excess oil.

Melt the remaining butter in the pan and cook the other half of the egg in the same manner.

Once both egg crepes are cooked, spread your mayonnaise over one side of each of them, add on the lettuce, tomato, avocado, and bacon. Roll them up like a burrito and enjoy!

KETO BLUEBERRY PANCAKES

These low-carb pancakes will remind you of all your favorite classic blueberry pancakes, but without the guilt! To keep these low-carb, you can enjoy them with fresh berries and whipped cream or Lakanto brand sugar-free maple-flavored syrup. These options are much lower in carbs than traditional maple syrup but just as delicious!

Details:

Number of Servings: **3**

Time Needed to Prepare: 3 minutes
Time Required to Cook: 10 minutes
Total Preparation/Cook Time: 13 minutes

Number of Calories in Individual Servings: 363
Protein Grams: 14
Fat Grams: 28
Total Carbohydrates Grams: 17
Net Carbohydrates Grams: 11

Ingredients:

- Eggs – 4
- Almond flour – 1.33 cup
- Almond milk – 3 tablespoons
- Vanilla extract - .5 teaspoon
- Baking powder – 2 teaspoons
- Sea salt - .25 teaspoon
- Swerve sugar-free sweetener – 1 tablespoon

- Blueberries - .75 cup
- Butter – 2 tablespoons

Instructions:

In a bowl, whisk together your eggs before adding in the almond flour, almond milk, vanilla extract, baking powder, and Swerve sweetener.

Once the batter is fully combined, gently fold in the blueberries, either fresh or frozen.

Heat a large electric griddle or a non-stick skillet over medium heat. Once hot, grease the skillet with the reserved butter and ladle the pancakes onto the pan. Each pancake should contain about .25 cups of batter.

Once the first side of the pancakes is cooked and golden, gently flip them over. Be careful not to mess with the pancakes while they are cooking. You only want to touch them when flipping.

Once both sides of the pancakes are cooked, remove them from the stove and serve them with fruit and whipped cream or Lakanto's sugar-free maple-flavored syrup.

KETO SAUSAGE AND CHEESE VEGETABLE FRITTATA

This frittata is full of breakfast sausage, vegetables, cream cheese, and cheddar cheese. You will love every slice of this delectable frittata, and even more than that, you will like how it gives you a week's worth of breakfast to store in the fridge or freezer to effortlessly enjoy.

Details:

Number of Servings: **8**

Time Needed to Prepare: 10 minutes
Time Required to Cook: 50 minutes
Total Preparation/Cook Time: 1 hour

Number of Calories in Individual Servings: 389
Protein Grams: 20
Fat Grams: 31
Total Carbohydrates Grams: 5
Net Carbohydrates Grams: 4

Ingredients:

- Eggs – 6
- Cream cheese, cut into cubes – 8 ounces
- Ground breakfast sausage – 1 pound
- Cheddar cheese, shredded – 8 ounces
- Kale, chopped – 1.5 cups
- Onion, small, diced – 1

- Bell pepper, diced – 1
- Garlic, minced – 3 cloves
- Half n' half - .5 cup
- Water - .5 cup

Instructions:

Preheat your oven to a temperature of Fahrenheit three-hundred and seventy-five degrees.

In a large skillet, which should be set to medium-high heat, add the breakfast sausage, onion, garlic, and bell pepper, and cook it until the sausage is browned all the way through. Drain off any excess fat after cooking.

Add the cream cheese to the skillet and stir it into the meat until it is fully melted. Place the chopped kale into the skillet, cover it with a lid, and then allow it to cook for an additional two minutes until it has reduced in size.

In a bowl, vigorously whisk together the eggs, half n' half, and water until the egg white proteins are fully broken down into the yolk and liquid.

Grease an eleven by seven-inch casserole dish and then add the sausage and vegetable mixture into it. Sprinkle the cheddar cheese over the top before pouring the egg mixture over everything.

Use a spoon to slightly move the ingredients around so the eggs get between all the vegetables and meat.

Place the casserole dish in the oven and allow it to cook until the center of the frittata is fully cooked for about forty minutes.

Remove the dish from the oven and allow it to cool for ten minutes before serving.

KETO CHEESE AND SAUSAGE SCONES

These scones are a fantastic way to enjoy the morning, whether you are relaxing at the dining room table or rushing out on the town. They are full of delicious cheddar cheese, breakfast sausage, sweet peppers, and onion for amazing flavor.

Details:

Number of Servings: **4**

Time Needed to Prepare: 5 minutes
Time Required to Cook: 10 minutes
Total Preparation/Cook Time: 15 minutes

Number of Calories in Individual Servings: 307
Protein Grams: 18
Fat Grams: 23
Total Carbohydrates Grams: 7
Net Carbohydrates Grams: 4

Ingredients:

- Eggs – 3
- Cheddar cheese, shredded – 1 cup
- Ground breakfast sausage – 4 ounces
- Almond flour - .75 cup
- Onion, diced - .5 cup
- Bell pepper, diced - .5 cup
- Sea salt - .5 teaspoon

- Black pepper, ground - .5 teaspoon

Instructions:

Preheat your oven to a temperature of Fahrenheit three-hundred and seventy-five degrees and prepare an aluminum baking sheet by lining it with either kitchen parchment or a silicone liner.

Place the breakfast sausage, bell pepper, and onion in a skillet and cook it all together over medium heat until the meat is cooked all the way through and the vegetables are soft. Remove it from the heat and allow it to cool.

In a bowl, mix the almond flour, black pepper, baking powder, and sea salt.

Into another bowl, combine the eggs and the cheese. Add this mixture to the almond flour mixture along with the cooled vegetables and sausage. Combine fully.

Using a large spoon, scoop out the dough into portions, with each scone containing about two tablespoons of dough. The mixture will be sticky, but place it on the pan the best as you can. Each dough portion should be placed about two inches apart. Slightly flatten the dough mounds with your fingers.

Place the scones in the oven until cooked all the way through and golden, about eight to ten minutes. Once done, allow the scones to cool for a few minutes before enjoying.

LUNCH

These simple meals are the perfect way to enjoy an afternoon. Whether you are at home, work, or on the go, you will find simple go-to solutions to eat healthy and delicious meals. You will find both meals that you can prepare ahead of time and store in the fridge to enjoy throughout the week and quick and simple meals to prepare at a moment's notice.

SHRIMP GREEK SALAD

This salad is satisfying and delicious, and it will keep you full and nourished all day long! Whether you are preparing to start your fast or break a fast, you will find that this is the perfect meal. With the fibrous brown rice, fresh vegetables, and refreshing shrimp, you will find this salad different from any other.

Details:

Number of Servings: **5**

Time Needed to Prepare: 10 minutes
Time Required to Cook: 0 minutes
Total Preparation/Cook Time: 10 minutes

Number of Calories in Individual Servings: 500
Protein Grams: 22
Fat Grams: 25
Total Carbohydrates Grams: 46
Net Carbohydrates Grams: 41

Ingredients:

- Brown rice, cooked – 4 cups
- Shrimp, medium, cooked – 1 pound
- Cucumber, diced – 1
- Roma tomatoes, diced – 2
- Parsley, chopped - .75 cup
- Scallions, thinly sliced – 3
- Kalamata olives pitted and chopped - .5 cup
- Feta cheese, crumbled – 6 ounces

- Olive oil - .33 cup
- Garlic, minced – 3 cloves
- Lemon juice – .33 cup
- Oregano, dried – 2 teaspoons
- Sea salt – 1 teaspoon

Instructions:

Add the cooked brown rice, shrimp, and vegetables together in a large salad bowl and toss them together.

In a smaller bowl, vigorously whisk together the olive oil, lemon juice, garlic, oregano, and sea salt until fully combined.

Pour the prepared vinaigrette over the tossed salad and once again toss to fully coat the salad in the vinaigrette. Carefully fold in the feta cheese to prevent it from falling apart.

Store the salad in the fridge for up to three to four days.

SWEET PEPPER NACHOS

Rather than fattening chips, these nachos are made with low-carb sweet bell peppers. You will love the bell peppers filled with taco-flavored beef, cheddar cheese, fresh tomatoes, cilantro, and sour cream. Of course, you can also add in any of your favorite nacho toppings to customize these to perfection.

The Details:

Number of Servings: **5**

Time Needed to Prepare: 10 minutes
Time Required to Cook: 15 minutes
Total Preparation/Cook Time: 25 minutes

Number of Calories in Individual Servings: 410
Protein Grams: 23
Fat Grams: 30
Total Carbohydrates Grams: 10
Net Carbohydrates Grams: 8

Ingredients:

- Bell peppers – 3
- Ground beef, 80/20 – 1 pound
- Cheddar cheese, shredded – 1 cup
- Chili powder – 1 teaspoon
- Sea salt – 1 teaspoon
- Onion powder - .5 teaspoon
- Cumin – 1 teaspoon
- Black pepper, ground - .5 teaspoon

- Garlic powder – .5 teaspoon
- Roma tomatoes, diced – 2
- Sour cream - .5 cup
- Cilantro, chopped - .5 cup

Instructions:

Slice around the top of the bell peppers so that you can cleanly remove the stems. Once the stems are removed, pull out the seeds and membrane. Slice each of the bell peppers into six portions that are shaped like boats or chips. Set the bell peppers aside.

Place the ground beef in a large skillet and cook it until it is fully cooked through. Drain off any excess fat and then stir in the diced tomatoes, chopped cilantro, chili powder, cumin, sea salt, black pepper, onion powder, and garlic powder.

Preheat the oven to a temperature of Fahrenheit three-hundred and seventy-five degrees and line an aluminum baking pan with either a silicone mat or kitchen parchment.

Place the bell pepper boats on the baking sheet and then fill them with the beef mixture. Top the beef off with the shredded cheese. Cook the bell pepper boats in the oven until hot and the cheese is melted about ten minutes.

Once the peppers are done cooking, top them with the sour cream and enjoy!

Optional: if you would like the bell peppers to be softer, you can place them in a glass baking dish with a few tablespoons of water, cover the dish with aluminum foil, and allow it to cook in the oven for fifteen minutes.

SPAGHETTI SQUASH GARLIC NOODLES WITH CHICKEN

These noodles are perfect for enjoying on-the-go, as they can be eaten either hot or cold. Simply pack up your noodles in a warm thermos or a cold bag with some ice, and you have a full nutritious meal ready to go. This means that even if you need to break your fast during the middle of your workday or while running errands, you will be prepared with a tasty and nutritious meal with little effort.

Details:

Number of Servings: **4**

Time Needed to Prepare: 10 minutes
Time Required to Cook: 25 minutes
Total Preparation/Cook Time: 35 minutes

Number of Calories in Individual Servings: 438
Protein Grams: 33
Fat Grams: 14
Total Carbohydrates Grams: 49
Net Carbohydrates Grams: 38

Ingredients:

- Spaghetti squash, 5 pounds, cooked – 1
- Zucchini, julienned – 1
- Red bell pepper, small, minced – 1
- Cilantro, chopped - .5 cup

- Almonds, toasted, chopped - .25 cup
- Soy sauce or coconut aminos replacement - .66 cup
- Coconut milk, full fat - .25 cup
- Garlic, minced – 6 cloves
- Ginger, grated – 2 tablespoons
- Red curry paste – 2 tablespoons
- Fish sauce or vegan replacement – 2 tablespoons
- Lakanto golden sugar-free monk fruit sweetener – 3 tablespoons
- Chicken thighs, chopped into 1-inch cubes – 1 pound

Instructions:

If your spaghetti squash is not already cooked, you can prepare it by chopping it in half lengthwise, removing the seeds, and then placing it facing upward on a baking sheet. Lightly brush the squash with oil and then cook it until tender (about twenty-five minutes) at a temperature of Fahrenheit four-hundred and fifty degrees.

Prepare the chicken by placing it in a large non-stick skillet over a temperature of medium-high heat and allow it to cook until fully cooked through about seven to nine minutes. The internal temperature of the chicken must reach one-hundred and sixty-five degrees Fahrenheit to avoid food poisoning. Set aside.

In a blender, combine the soy sauce, coconut milk, garlic, ginger, red curry paste, fish sauce, and Lakanto sweetener until no chunks are remaining.

Run a fork through the hot spaghetti squash to form noodles out of the flesh. Transfer the "noodles" to a large bowl and toss them together with the cooked chicken, blended sauce, cilantro, zucchini, red bell pepper, and almonds.

Serve the noodles hot or cold. Store in the fridge for five to six days.

KETO CALIFORNIA ROLL BOWLS

Even if you are eating a low-carb/keto diet, you can still enjoy your favorite California rolls with these delicious bowls! They are full of protein from the crab, along with other important nutrients from the cauliflower rice, avocado, cucumber, nori, and sesame seeds. Your favorite food is now healthier than ever!

Details:

Number of Servings: **2**

Number of Calories in Individual Servings: 310
Protein Grams: 19
Fat Grams: 20
Total Carbohydrates Grams: 13
Net Carbohydrates Grams: 6

Ingredients:

- Cauliflower rice – 1.5 cups
- Avocado, thinly sliced - .5
- Cucumber, thinly sliced – 1
- Scallions, thinly sliced – 1
- Nori sheet, cut into small pieces - .5
- Crabmeat, canned – 6 ounces
- Seasoned rice vinegar – 1 tablespoon
- White sesame seeds, toasted - .5 tablespoon
- Black sesame seeds, toasted - .5 tablespoon
- Mayonnaise – 2 tablespoons
- Sriracha sauce – 2 teaspoons

Instructions:

In a bowl, whisk together the sriracha sauce and mayonnaise until they are fully combined and then set aside.

Steam the cauliflower rice in the microwave or on the stove until it is tender. Once done cooking, stir in the rice vinegar.

Divide the cooked cauliflower rice between two bowls and top it with the cucumbers, avocado, scallions, and crab meat. Drizzle the sriracha mayonnaise over the top and then sprinkle on the sesame seeds.

Enjoy the bowls immediately or store them in the fridge for up to three days before enjoying. Wait to add the chopped nori until immediately before serving so that it remains crispy.

KETO CHICKEN AVOCADO SALAD

This chicken salad is one of the most flavorful you will ever taste, with mashed avocado and Ranch dressing in place of mayonnaise, and with added bacon and cheddar cheese. This chicken salad can be served with your favorite low-carb snacking options or butterhead lettuce, as used in the recipe.

Details:

Number of Servings: **4**

Time Needed to Prepare: 5 minutes
Time Required to Cook: 0 minutes
Total Preparation/Cook Time: 5 minutes

Number of Calories in Individual Servings: 434
Protein Grams: 32
Fat Grams: 29
Total Carbohydrates Grams: 9
Net Carbohydrates Grams: 4

Ingredients:

- Chicken, cooked, diced – 2 cups
- Avocado, lightly mashed – 1
- Bacon, cooked, chopped – 6 slices
- Sea salt – 1 teaspoon
- Cheddar cheese, shredded - .75 cup
- Celery, diced - .75 cup

- Scallions, thinly sliced - .75 cup
- Primal Kitchen's Ranch or Caesar dressing - .25 cup
- Black pepper, ground - .25 teaspoon
- Butter lettuce – 2 heads

Instructions:

In a large bowl, toss together all ingredients, except the lettuce, until fully combined and coated in the dressing. Taste and adjust the seasonings to taste, add more dressing if desired.

Serve immediately with the butter lettuce or save in the fridge for up to five days.

DINNER

Whether you are craving your favorite comfort food or a full meal that you can share with the whole family, you will love these healthy and delicious dinners that are perfect for enjoying before beginning an overnight fast.

BIG MAC SALAD BOWL

No matter how delicious and nutritious food might be, we all have our guilty pleasures. One of these comfort foods for many people is the Big Mac burger. However, you can allow yourself to enjoy all the flavors of this favorite meal without the fattening ingredients that will leave you feeling bloated and sluggish. This version of the Big Mac is full of all your favorite ingredients but without the unhealthy additives. You can enjoy this low-carb/keto Big Mac, while still gaining health and losing weight.

While it may be typical to use full-fat meats on the ketogenic diet, in this recipe, you want to use lean ground beef. Otherwise, the burger will be overly greasy. Trust me; it's perfect this way.

Details:

Number of Servings: **4**

Time Needed to Prepare: 7 minutes
Time Required to Cook: 7 minutes
Total Preparation/Cook Time: 14 minutes

Number of Calories in Individual Servings: 525
Protein Grams: 30
Fat Grams: 41
Total Carbohydrates Grams: 5
Net Carbohydrates Grams: 4

Ingredients:

- Ground beef, lean – 1 pound

- Black pepper, ground – 1 teaspoon
- Onion, sliced in rounds - .5 cup
- Cheddar cheese, shredded – 1 cup
- Sea salt – 1 teaspoon
- Pickles, sliced - .25 cup
- Iceberg lettuce, chopped – 4 cups
- Yellow mustard – 4 teaspoons
- Mayonnaise - .5 cup
- Vinegar – 2 teaspoons
- Lakanto monk fruit sweetener – 1.5 teaspoons
- Pickles, diced – 4 teaspoons
- Onion, finely minced – 1 tablespoon
- Paprika, smoked - .25 teaspoon

Instructions:

Begin by making your special sauce. To do this, whisk together the mustard, mayonnaise, vinegar, sweetener, diced pickles, minced onion, and smoked paprika. Set the sauce aside to allow the flavors to meld together. The sauce can be made up to a week in advance, and it tastes even better after resting overnight in the fridge.

Heat a large skillet over a temperature of medium heat and brown the ground beef. Once it is mostly cooked with only a little pink remaining add in the sea salt and black pepper, and then finish cooking it until the pink disappears, and it is cooked all the way through.

Divide the lettuce, pickles, onions, and cheese evenly between four bowls, and then add the browned beef on top. By placing the hot beef on top of the other ingredients, you will melt the cheese.

Drizzle the special sauce over the top of the Big Mac bowls and serve immediately.

"STUFFED" CABBAGE CASSEROLE

This low-carb "stuffed" cabbage casserole is much easier to make than traditional stuffed cabbage, as you simply layer everything in the pan and allow the flavors to meld together.

Details:

Number of Servings: **5**

Time Needed to Prepare: 5 minutes
Time Required to Cook: 25 minutes
Total Preparation/Cook Time: 30 minutes

Number of Calories in Individual Servings: 398
Protein Grams: 26
Fat Grams: 24
Total Carbohydrates Grams: 20
Net Carbohydrates Grams: 14

Ingredients:

- Ground beef, 85/15 – 1 pound
- Olive oil – 1 tablespoon
- Bell pepper, orange, sliced – 1
- Sweet onion, sliced – 1
- Garlic, minced – 3 cloves
- Diced tomatoes – 1 can
- Sea salt – 1 teaspoon
- Smoked paprika - .5 teaspoon

- Garlic powder - .5 teaspoon
- Dried oregano – .5 teaspoon
- Onion powder - .5 teaspoon
- Black pepper, ground - .5 teaspoon
- Green cabbage, chopped – 1 head
- Cheddar cheese, shredded – 1 cup

Instructions:

To a large skillet over medium-high heat, add the olive oil, ground beef, bell pepper, and onion. Allow the vegetables and meat to cook together until the beef is mostly browned. Add in the garlic and cook until the meat is fully cooked.

Into the skillet, add the canned tomatoes and seasonings, stirring the ingredients all together. Add the cabbage to the top of the skillet, cover the skillet with a lid, and cook until the cabbage is tender about fifteen minutes.

Sprinkle the cheese over the top of the dish and place the lid back on top for a couple of minutes, until the cheese is melted. Serve immediately and store any leftovers in the fridge for up to five or six days.

KETO CHILI

This low-carb chili is full of flavor and seasoning, complete with a touch of cocoa powder to deepen and meld the flavors together. Not only can you cook this chili on the stove for a quick meal, you can also cook it in a slow cooker for even deeper flavors, and an easy meal prepared ahead of time.

Details:

Number of Servings: **8**

Time Needed to Prepare: 5 minutes
Time Required to Cook: 40 minutes
Total Preparation/Cook Time: 45 minutes

Number of Calories in Individual Servings: 307
Protein Grams: 25
Fat Grams: 18
Total Carbohydrates Grams: 12
Net Carbohydrates Grams: 9

Ingredients:

- Ground beef, 85/15 – 2 pounds
- Jalapeno, seeds removed and diced – 1
- Bell pepper, diced – 1
- Beef broth – 32 ounces
- Tomato sauce – 15 ounces
- Tomatoes with green chilies – 10 ounces

- Tomato paste – 7 ounces
- Sea salt – 2 teaspoons
- Garlic, minced – 4 cloves
- Chili powder – 2 tablespoons
- Cocoa powder – 2 teaspoons
- Garlic powder – 1 teaspoon
- Cumin – 1 teaspoon
- Oregano, dried – 1 teaspoon
- Black pepper, ground - .5 teaspoon

Instructions:

In a large Dutch oven or pot brown the ground beef. Once fully cooked, drain off any excess fat.

Add the remaining ingredients and stir them all together until fully combined. Simmer the chili over low heat for thirty minutes, until the sauce has thickened and reduced. Serve immediately or store in the fridge for up to a week.

Alternatively, after browning the beef, you can combine all the ingredients in a slow cooker and then allow it to cook on low for four hours or high for two hours.

CREAMY ARTICHOKE SPINACH SOUP

This creamy soup is just like your favorite artichoke and spinach dip but without the guilt! You can now enjoy it low-carb for a complete meal, and any occasion!

Details:

Number of Servings: **6**

Time Needed to Prepare: 5 minutes
Time Required to Cook: 22 minutes
Total Preparation/Cook Time: 27 minutes

Number of Calories in Individual Servings: 440
Protein Grams: 12
Fat Grams: 37
Total Carbohydrates Grams: 17
Net Carbohydrates Grams: 12

Ingredients:

- Frozen Spinach, chopped – 9 ounces
- Artichoke hearts, canned and drained, chopped – 14 ounces
- Chicken broth – 4 cups
- Heavy cream – 1 cup
- Cream cheese – 8 ounces
- Parmesan cheese, grated – 1 cup
- Garlic, minced – 4 cloves

- Sea salt – 1 teaspoon
- Onion, diced – 1
- Butter – 2 tablespoons
- Black pepper, ground - .5 teaspoon

Instructions:

In a large Dutch oven or pot, melt the butter and then add in the onion, cooking it until slightly softened about five minutes. Add in the garlic and cook for one to two more minutes.

Add the spinach to the Dutch oven and allow it to thaw and cook until warmed through, about five to seven minutes, and then stir in the sea salt and black pepper.

Add the artichoke hearts and chicken broth to the pot and then allow it to heat about five to ten additional minutes.

Reduce the heat to low before adding in the cream cheese and heavy cream. Melt the cream cheese slowly, being careful not to curdle the cream. Stir in the Parmesan cheese.

Serve the soup immediately or store it in the fridge for up to six days.

DESSERT

KETO CHOCOLATE MOUSSE

This chocolate mousse only takes a few minutes to whip up and can be enjoyed immediately. Serve it as-is or pour it into a low-carb keto pie crust for a chocolate mousse pie.

Details:

Number of Servings: **4**

Time Needed to Prepare: 5 minutes
Time Required to Cook: 0 minutes
Total Preparation/Cook Time: 5 minutes

Number of Calories in Individual Servings: 324
Protein Grams: 3
Fat Grams: 34
Total Carbohydrates Grams: 6
Net Carbohydrates Grams: 4

Ingredients:

- Cocoa powder – .33 cup
- Lakanto monk fruit sweetener – 2 tablespoons
- Heavy whipping cream – 1.5 cups

Instructions:

Place the heavy cream in a bowl and use a hand mixer or stand mixer to beat it on medium speed.

Once the cream begins to thicken, add the monk fruit sweetener and cocoa and continue to beat it until stiff peaks form.

Serve the mousse immediately or store it in the fridge for up to twenty-four hours before enjoying it. If desired, you can serve it with Lily's stevia-sweetened chocolate for chunks.

NO-BAKE PEANUT BUTTER PIE

This pie is the perfect treat to serve at the holidays, at a potluck, or any other time you might be craving a sweet treat. No matter the occasion, you will find that this creamy no-bake peanut butter pie will offer you all the sweetness and flavor you are craving. If you want, you can even drizzle melted Lily's stevia-sweetened chocolate over the top.

Details:

Number of Servings: **8**

Time Needed to Prepare: 15 minutes
Time Required to Cook: 0 minutes
Total Preparation/Cook Time: 15 minutes

Number of Calories in Individual Servings: 518
Protein Grams: 12
Fat Grams: 49
Total Carbohydrates Grams: 12
Net Carbohydrates Grams: 9

Ingredients:

- Almond flour – 1 cup
- Butter softened – 2 tablespoons
- Vanilla - .5 teaspoon
- Lakanto monk fruit sweetener – 1.5 tablespoons
- Cocoa powder – 3 tablespoons
- Cream cheese softened – 16 ounces
- Heavy cream – .75 cup

- Vanilla – 2 teaspoons
- Swerve confectioner's sweetener - .66 cup
- Peanut butter or Sun Butter, unsweetened – .75 cup

Instructions:

Combine the almond flour, butter, .5 teaspoon of vanilla, Lakanto sweetener, and cocoa powder in a bowl with a fork until it forms a crumbly mixture. Press this mixture into a nine-inch pie plate and then allow it to chill in the fridge while you prepare the filling.

In a large bowl, beat together the cream cheese, peanut butter, confectioners Swerve, and remaining vanilla until light and creamy. Using a spatula scrape down the sides of the bowl before adding in the heavy cream.

Beat the filling some more until the heavy cream is incorporated and the mixture is once again light and creamy.

Pour the filling into the prepared crust and allow it to chill for two hours before serving. Slice and enjoy.

BERRIES WITH RICOTTA CREAM

This dessert is simple and quick to make with healthy fresh ingredients, making it the perfect treat year-round. However, it is especially delicious in the spring, when berries are in season.

Details:

Number of Servings: **4**

Time Needed to Prepare: 5 minutes
Time Required to Cook: 0 minutes
Total Preparation/Cook Time: 5 minutes

Number of Calories in Individual Servings: 217
Protein Grams: 11
Fat Grams: 15
Total Carbohydrates Grams: 9
Net Carbohydrates Grams: 7

Ingredients:

- Ricotta, whole milk – 1.5 cups
- Heavy cream – 2 tablespoons
- Lemon zest – 1.5 teaspoons
- Swerve confectioner's sweetener – .25 cup
- Vanilla extract – 1 teaspoon
- Blackberries - .5 cup
- Raspberries - .5 cup
- Blueberries - .5 cup

Instructions:

In a large bowl, add all of the ingredients, except for the berries, and whip them together with a hand mixer until completely smooth.

Set out four parfait glasses and divide half of the berries between all of them. Top the berries with half of the ricotta mixture, the remaining half of the berries, and lastly, the second half of the ricotta mixture.

Serve the parfaits immediately or within the next twenty-four hours.

Conclusion

Thank you for purchasing this book, and congratulations on finishing *Intermittent Fasting for Women Over 50*! I hope that through the pages of this book, you were able to gain the knowledge, understanding, and confidence you need to succeed with losing weight and gaining improved health.

While intermittent fasting may be an unorthodox lifestyle at this point, for centuries, it was a standard and everyday part of life worldwide. Not only that, but science has proven it to be both safe and effective. There is no reason to hold back from this positive lifestyle that has proven through both time and science to be such an improvement. You have everything to gain and nothing to lose by taking a step forward and making a change for the better. Whether you choose to practice intermittent fasting alone or with the ketogenic diet, you can expect to experience many benefits. While it may take a little time to adjust to the change in lifestyle, as all changes do, take heart in knowing that within a month, most people adjust and adapt.

The recipes at the end of this book will help you to stay full, satisfied, and nourished not only during your eating windows, but also your fasting windows. They are simple to follow, yet full of flavor that will keep you coming back to the dishes time and again.

You are now armed with everything you need to succeed on the road to intermittent fasting. There is no reason to hesitate. The sooner you begin, the sooner you can expect results.

Finally, if you found this book useful in any way, a review on Amazon is always appreciated!

Made in the USA
Coppell, TX
22 December 2019